# PATENTS

## THE EXPERIENCE
## OF ILLNESS

For Jill and Julie

# PATIENTS

## THE EXPERIENCE OF ILLNESS

by Mark L. Rosenberg, M.D.

Introduction by Robert Coles, M.D.

THE SAUNDERS PRESS

W. B. Saunders Company

Philadelphia • London • Toronto

THE SAUNDERS PRESS/SAUNDERS PAPERBACKS
W. B. Saunders Company
West Washington Square
Philadelphia, PA 19105

IN THE UNITED STATES
DISTRIBUTED TO THE TRADE BY
HOLT, RINEHART AND WINSTON
383 Madison Avenue
New York, New York 10017

IN CANADA
DISTRIBUTED BY
HOLT, RINEHART AND WINSTON, LTD.
55 Horner Avenue
Toronto, Ontario
M8Z 4X6
Canada

**Library of Congress Cataloging in Publication Data**

Rosenberg, Mark L   1945-
Patients, the experience of illness.

1. Sick—Psychology.   2. Sick—Interviews.
3. Hospital patients—Interviews.   I. Title.
[DNLM:   1. Medicine—Case studies.   2. Medicine—
Pictorial works.   WB293 R813p]
R726.5.R67   155.9'16   79-67115

Published simultaneously in hardcover and paperback.

Library of Congress Catalog Card Number: 79-67115
W. B. Saunders Company ISBN: 0-7216-7702-9 paperback
0-7216-7701-0 hardcover
Holt, Rinehart and Winston ISBN: 0-03-056742-4 paperback
0-03-056743-2 hardcover

Print Number 9 8 7 6 5 4 3 2

First Edition

# Acknowledgments

I want to thank those people who shared with me parts of their lives as patients, family, friends, or care-givers. I appreciate their trust in me and their giving of themselves. I am grateful to the physicians and clinicians who helped select the patients for this study and allowed me to observe them and discuss the medical care they rendered: Drs. William Boger, John Collins, Joan Fluri, David Fromm, Stuart Goldman, Louis Caplan, Robert Petersen, Chester Rosoff, Lowell Schnipper, and Ted Steinman; Libby Battit and Regina Bowler, nurse-clinicians.

I am also indebted to those institutions which allowed me access to their facilities and patients. My thanks go to Dr. Mitchell Rabkin, of the Beth Israel Hospital, Dr. William Hassan, Jr. of the Peter Bent Brigham Hospital, Mr. David Weiner of the Childrens' Hospital Medical Center, Mr. Paul Schulman of the Lemuel Shattuck Hospital, Dr. Joseph Dorsey of the Harvard Community Health Plan, Mr. Carlton Smith of the Veterans Administration Medical Center, and Dr. J. Michael Lazarus of the Kidney Center.

Many people encouraged me and supported me in this work. In particular I am grateful to Dr. Howard Hiatt who allowed me to devote time to this project while I was teaching at the Harvard School of Public Health. Mr. Robert Simone taught my only formal photography course and both he and the photographers of Nexus encouraged me in my photographic endeavors. Dr. Mark Field introduced me to the field of medical sociology and provided helpful comments on the manuscript. The Charles E. Merrill Fund and the Commonwealth Fund provided financial support for work in this book.

Ms. Laurie Pearlman provided valuable editorial assistance and with Ms. Lauren Goldberg helped to prepare and assemble the material into its final form.

Throughout the three years I worked on this book, my wife, Jill Dimond, provided encouragement, emotional support, and helpful criticism. Her judgement, sensitivity, and firm editorial hand made a world of difference.

MARK L. ROSENBERG

# Contents

# Introduction

## by Robert Coles, M.D.

I remember going on house-calls with William Carlos Williams. I wrote an undergraduate thesis on his poetry, became acquainted with him, and as a medical student, was invited to see that other, important side of his life, the daily visits he made to the sick, the hurt, the lame—the mostly poor and immigrant families he looked after, day in and day out, with conscientious intelligence, with humor, and with empathy. As we climbed one set of stairs after another, he couldn't help giving me advice, pointing things out, offering the enthusiastic, pungent wisdom that always seemed in great supply and at the tip of his tongue. One day he became as brief as possible: "Doctors should keep their mouths shut more than they do—including me! We should look more; we should listen more. Patients are our teachers." Then he shut up and for the life of me, I couldn't get that usually talkative old doc going again for many minutes. Every time I came up with a starter, he pointed—at something to be seen, at some people who were speaking to each other. Only when we got off Paterson's busy streets, and back into his car, did he resume his usual self, so to speak—with an explanation: "We've got to learn to stop ourselves; we've got to learn to surrender to 'them'—to our patients. They have stories to tell, too—lines of poetry in them; bad dreams and good ones; pictures to give us—of their wounds, and their smiles, and the deep worry-lines on their faces."

I thought of Dr. Williams as I went through this splendid book, which provides a touching evocation, really, of his spirit. He was a poet with a remarkably visual sense; he was a doctor. In this book a doctor, able to use a camera with sensitivity and restraint, brings us the words of ordinary, hard-pressed human beings, who are struggling, as we all do, to make sense of the world, including its arbitrariness—the diseases that visit us, out of nowhere it seems, and eventually (one or more of them) take us away for good. Again and again when I was in medical school, Dr. Williams kept urging me to "get out" into various neighborhoods, to "go see," to "go hear," to let "them" be my guides. A book such as this is spiritual kin of Dr. Williams' writing. Mark Rosenberg has responded to the essence of his job—drawing from it these continuing encounters with men and women and children who for brief or long spells get called "patients."

Needless to say, we are all headed for such an "existential" situation, and one only hopes and prays that we will pass honorable muster—be as humble, as wry, as stoic, as *patient*, as some of the "patients" we get to meet in the course of our clinical work. Here are a few of "them"; here are some of us—fellow human beings; they are attentively seen and closely, respectfully heeded by a young physician who needs no admonitions from anyone about the importance of connecting the traditions of the humanities to medicine. His camera, his storyteller's ear, help us become a little more aware of what we may sometimes fail to notice: the looks of resignation, of suffering, the sounds of one person after another trying to come to terms with life's relentless, messy challenges, which may threaten to break us, but (psychologically, spiritually) can also become the making of us—until we once and for all leave. I hope many, many of us, and especially medical students and nursing students, get to meet Mark Rosenberg's "patients," and thereby get not only closer to themselves as future doctors or nurses, but as men and women given a special trust—to observe life in its most exposed, vulnerable and significant moments.

# Author's Introduction

As a physician, I had ordered hundreds of X-rays, but I had not fully appreciated what such an order could mean for a patient. Then, one Christmas Eve, I spent three hours in the hospital with a patient, Kay Finn, who had breast cancer that had spread to her bones and caused any movement to be extremely painful. I watched her that evening as she was transferred onto a steel stretcher, left waiting in the basement hall, transferred onto the X-ray table, and finally was returned to her bed three hours later. Her experience was worlds apart from that of the physician who had written and signed the X-ray order in ten seconds. I realized my medical training had given me no idea of what it was like to be a patient.

Certainly a patient's concern with his or her illness is not limited to the duration of the encounter with the physician. But it was only by spending many hours with each patient that I came to realize the extent to which an illness could pervade and change one's life. Within the brief time allocated to most doctor-patient encounters, however, even the most articulate patients often cannot communicate their concerns very effectively.

Each patient had his or her own way of dealing with illness. As a result, each chapter in this book is as much a portrait of a particular individual as it is the story of a particular disease. I was impressed by the strength these patients displayed. Though at times their strength appeared extraordinary, they were ordinary people who had been selected not for their strength, but for their willingness to talk. Perhaps this willingness to talk was a sign of that strength.

These patients were ordinary people with common diseases. Heart disease, cancer, and stroke are the leading causes of death for all Americans. And while it is uncommon for a stroke to occur in someone as young as Joel Bruinooge, his youth simply highlights the consequences of that illness. Almost one out of every twenty children born in this country has crossed eyes. One out of every ten to thirteen American women develops breast cancer. And each year, more than 44,000 Americans undergo kidney transplants or dialysis as treatment for end-stage renal disease.

Yet as common as these diseases are, the average person knows little about them. In our ignorance, we may think these diseases are more disabling and more disfiguring than they really are. In our culture, there are very few ways to correct such misimpressions. Pictures of sick people are conspicuous by their absence, and the segregation of sick people into hospitals and nursing homes ensures that most of us will never see "the real thing." An unfortunate consequence of always keeping illness under wraps is that we might come to think that sick people are too horrifying to look at. And if we can't look at them, we certainly can't talk to them. In the end, we may leave patients unable to talk about their illnesses with family or friends just when they are most in need of support.

I was particularly concerned about whether my photographing these patients made their experience with illness more difficult. Certainly, standing before a camera can make one acutely self-conscious. But being conscious of one's self and one's appearance need not be disturbing. How the subject feels depends, in part, on how the observer and subject interact, and this shows up in the photograph. These photographs reflect relationships that evolved over time. Sometimes these relationships became quite close, especially after we had spent time together during some particularly difficult or painful experiences. Yet despite this closeness, there were times when patients did not want to talk to me or be photographed. Three months after we had met, Kay Finn decided that she did not want to continue meeting with me. In fact, from that point on, she also chose not to meet with any friends or family members except her sister. This withdrawal was probably part of her preparation for death, which came four weeks later. On the other hand, when I asked Jeanne MacLaughlin how she felt about having been photographed during a difficult period, she replied: "At the moment, I had been feeling very rejected, and with your support and your interest, you lessened that feeling of rejection to some degree…because you were a man and you were not afraid to look at me. I could not understand why my husband was. It just helped. I can't explain why or how, but it did help." She seemed to be saying something which was confirmed by other patients as well: we can all give something valuable to someone who is ill by being willing to see and willing to hear. Then, perhaps, we can begin to understand more fully what the experience of illness can mean.

*This project began as an attempt to use photographs and tape-recorded interviews to show what it is like to be a patient and to receive medical care. I wanted to focus on people with common but serious diseases. To carry out this project, I first secured permission from the administrators and the Human Studies Committees of several different hospitals. I then asked individual physicians to select patients who might be interested in being photographed and in talking about their illness. Physicians explained to these patients that they were under no obligation to participate, that I would follow them as an observer and not as a physician, and that they could withdraw from the project at any time. All of the patients, except Kay Finn (who died before completion of the project), reviewed the material before it was printed; none had any hesitation about publishing this material or using real names.*

MARK L. ROSENBERG, M.D.

# Jenny Monroe

Jenny Monroe had crossed eyes—probably from the time of her birth. When she was seven years old she underwent surgery to correct the muscle balance and straighten her left eye. Jenny's mother stayed with her in the hospital for the three days and two nights of her hospitalization. Jenny's father, a physician, visited her in the hospital on the day of her surgery.

Jenny's eye doctor expects that her eyes will continue to correct themselves gradually over the next several years. Because of this, he did not correct her eyes completely. Jenny will continue to wear glasses until this self-correction is completed.

JENNY MONROE:
*My eye is crooked. It's been like that since I was about two years old...and now I'm seven. My teacher noticed it first and she said to my mother, "Why don't you look at her eye?"*

July 14, 1979

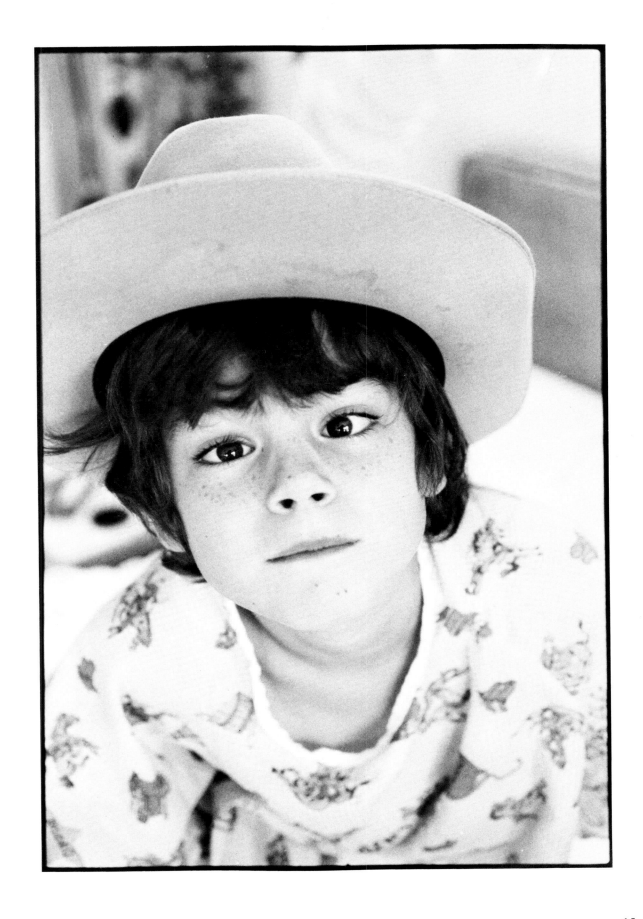

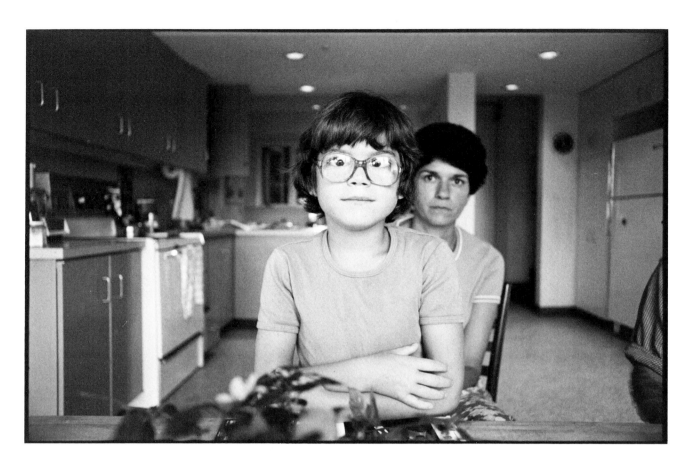

MRS. MONROE:
*When I was told she needed glasses I said, "Oh, my God!" And Dr. Petersen said immediately, "Well, if you think that, imagine what she's going to think!"*

October 21, 1979

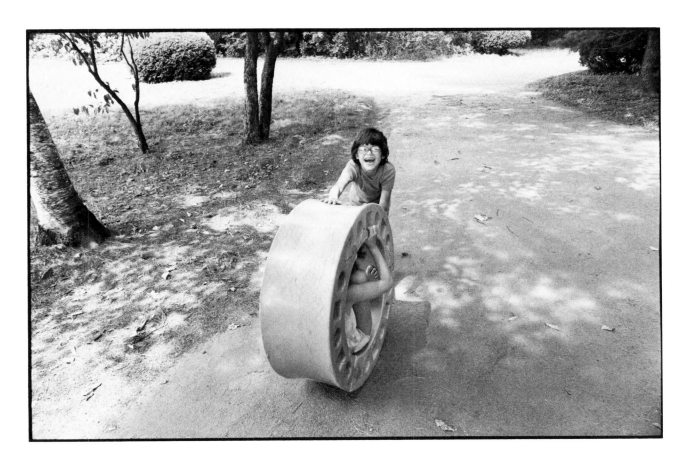

JENNY MONROE:
*It doesn't bother me or keep me from playing. But my friends
always ask me. "Why do you have glasses?" and I say,
"Because my eye's crooked." I even sort of forget I'm wearing
glasses...but most of the time I take them off because they're a
nuisance. They could get lost.*

July 14, 1979

*Sometimes people say mean things like, "Oh, Hi, four eyes." But
in school they don't say anything because there are people in my
class with glasses. So I'm not the only one. I think everybody has
a different thing, like a different kind of eye.*

August 9, 1979

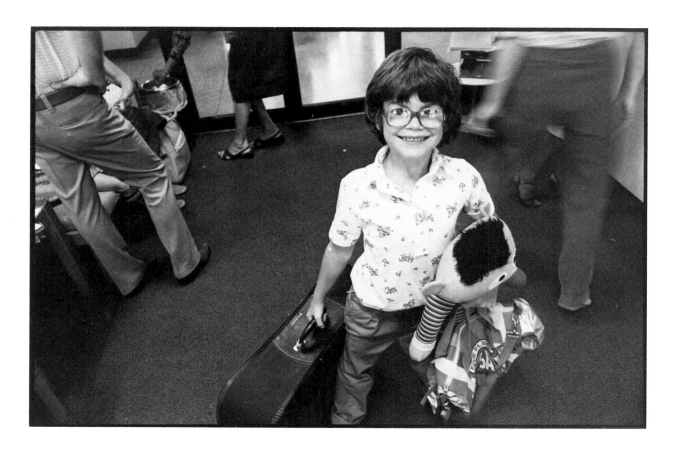

JENNY MONROE:
*My eye is going to be straightened out! I'm going into the hospital and the next day I'm going to have an operation, and then I'm going to go home. I'm really excited because I'm going to get a lot of presents and have a lot of ice cream. I'm sort of excited and sort of scared.*

July 14, 1979

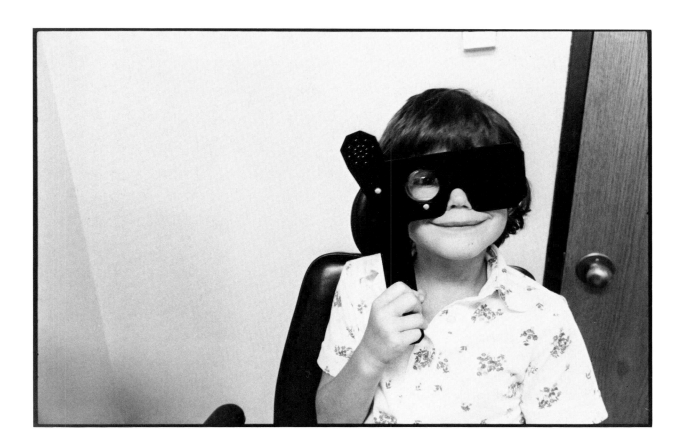

JENNY MONROE:
*I went to the eye clinic today and they told me everything that will happen to me tomorrow—they're going to straighten out my eye! And they told me what I can't do: I can't go swimming, I can't stick my finger in my eye, I can't drink tonight, and tomorrow I can't have breakfast.*

*After I wake up I might feel sick and I might throw up.*

July 16, 1979

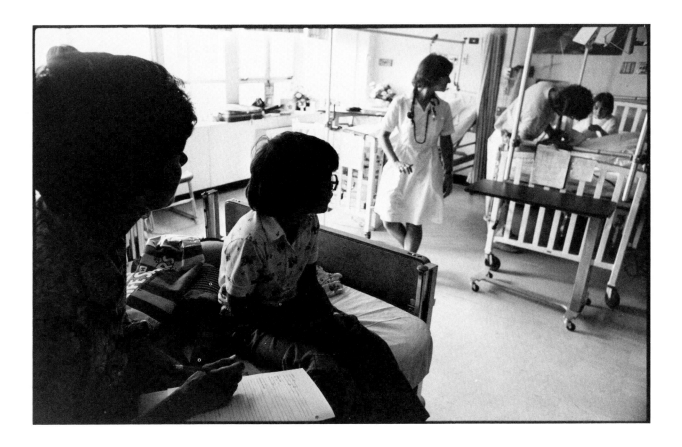

MRS. MONROE:
*We've tried to prepare her as much as possible for going into the hospital. She knows as much as we do because she was right there from the beginning when Dr. Petersen talked about it. Now we have some questions about the outcome.*

July 17, 1979

DR. PETERSEN:
*Although the risk of a healthy child having some serious complication from general anesthesia is probably less than 1 in 10,000, the thought is always in the back of a parent's mind that their child might be that one. That explanation makes me uncomfortable, so I guess it would probably make them uncomfortable too. But...I think the parents' decision about whether to let the child have the procedure has to be made knowing that there is a risk involved.*

July 16, 1979

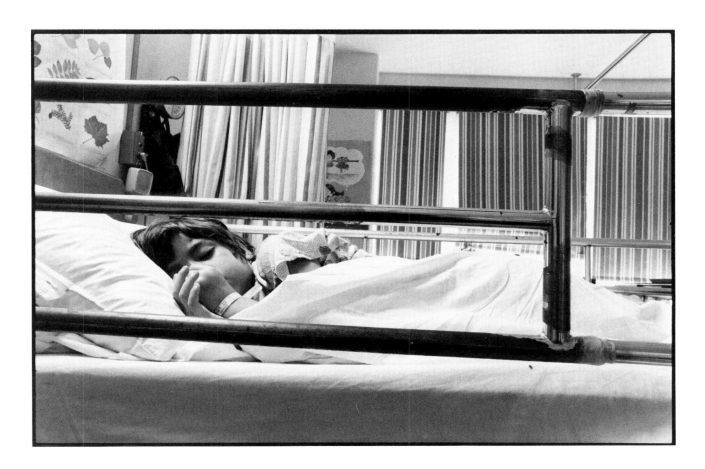

MRS. MONROE:
*Because of the possibility of being sued they tell
you there is a chance that something could go
wrong with the anesthesia, or the eye might
overcorrect itself. But I don't need to be told
that again and again—it's as if the doctor is pro-
tecting himself and not the patient.*

July 17, 1979

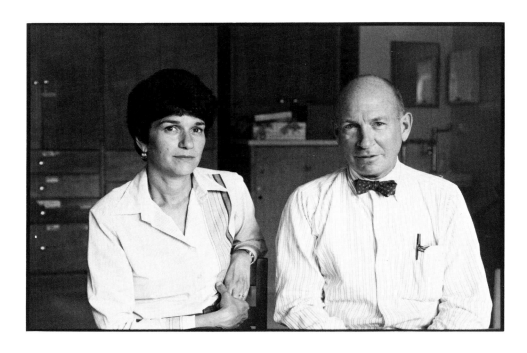

DR. MONROE:

*You can never give patients all they need and you can never tell them enough to satisfy them—it's a bottomless pit. When you do tell them something, their fear, anxiety, or pain is apt to make them forget it. So you'll just have to tell them again. They just crave information.*

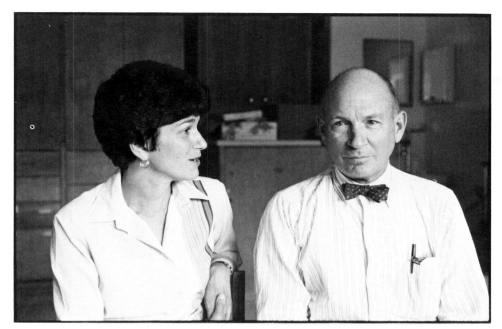

MRS. MONROE:

*That's a lot of baloney. It's that kind of thinking that leads doctors to give patients brief explanations that are unsatisfying, or maybe no explanations at all. Doctors think that as long as they know the reason, it doesn't have to be told to the patient. But the patient is entitled to know what's going on, and to know how to get in touch with the doctor when he's needed. In my case, for example, even though I'm married to a physician, I have never called Dr. Petersen during the whole time Jenny has been coming to him—I'd be terrified to call him, afraid he'd make me feel my questions weren't worth calling him away from his work.*

July 16, 1979

MRS. MONROE:

*What I'm really asking for is assurance—and I rarely feel I get it from a doctor.*

July 16, 1979

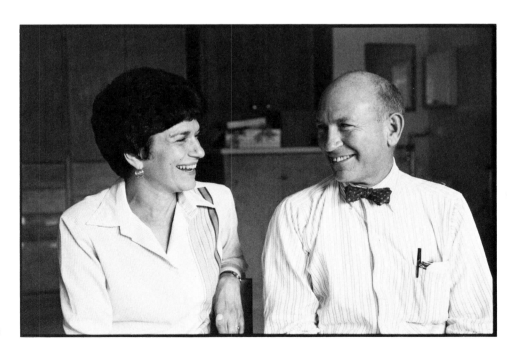

DR. MONROE:
*I'm not particularly apprehensive about it. I took the day off to come here because Jenny and my wife need a little support at this time. I was a physician on the staff here for 12 years so I know the hospital well and have quite a bit of confidence in it. I saw to it that Jenny was treated at the best local institution by very good people.*

July 17, 1979

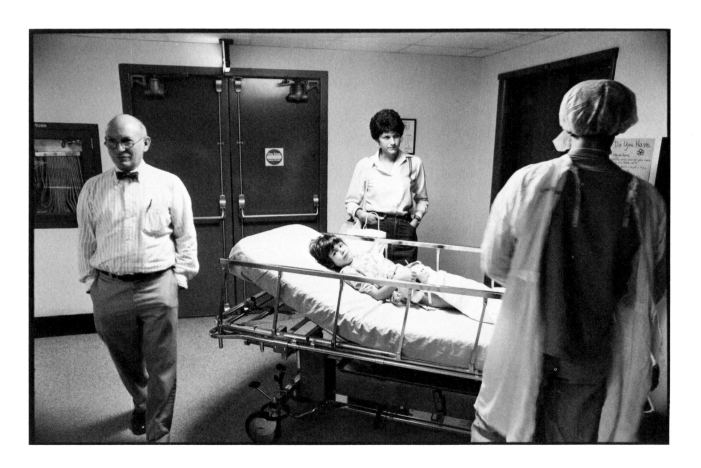

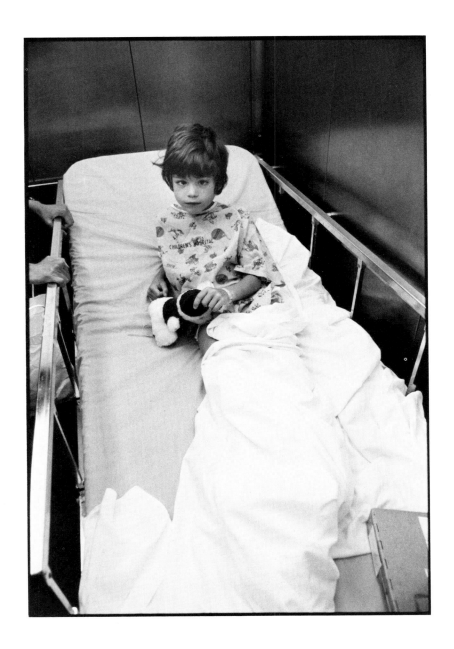

DR. MONROE:

She has a convergent strabismus and she will have this corrected. Her acuity in both eyes is quite good now but without the surgery she would tend to abandon one eye in favor of the other and the acuity in that abandoned eye would become very poor. By early adulthood she would see with only one eye; binocular vision would be gone. If she doesn't have binocular vision certain aspects of the world will escape her—sports will be more difficult, hitting a moving ball will be more difficult. Binocular vision and cosmetic improvement, these are the two things that interest me the most.

July 14, 1979

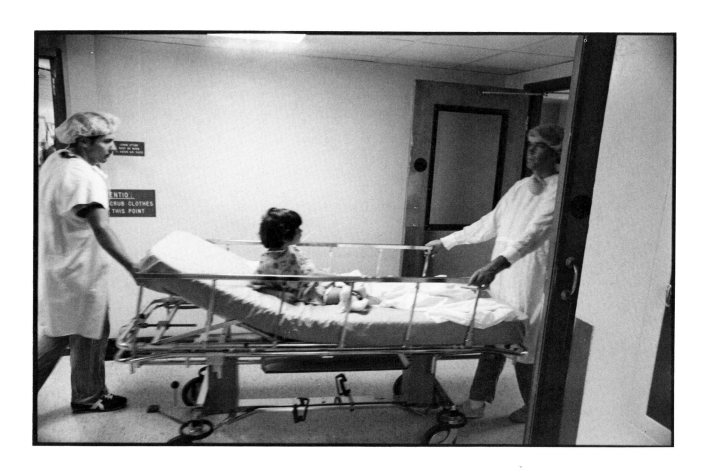

JENNY MONROE:
*Do you ever make a mistake when you operate?*

DR. PETERSEN:
*Yes, I do...but not very often.*

JENNY MONROE:
*If anything came out wrong, could I be blind?*

DR. PETERSEN:
*There's no way that that could happen, Jenny.*

July 16, 1979

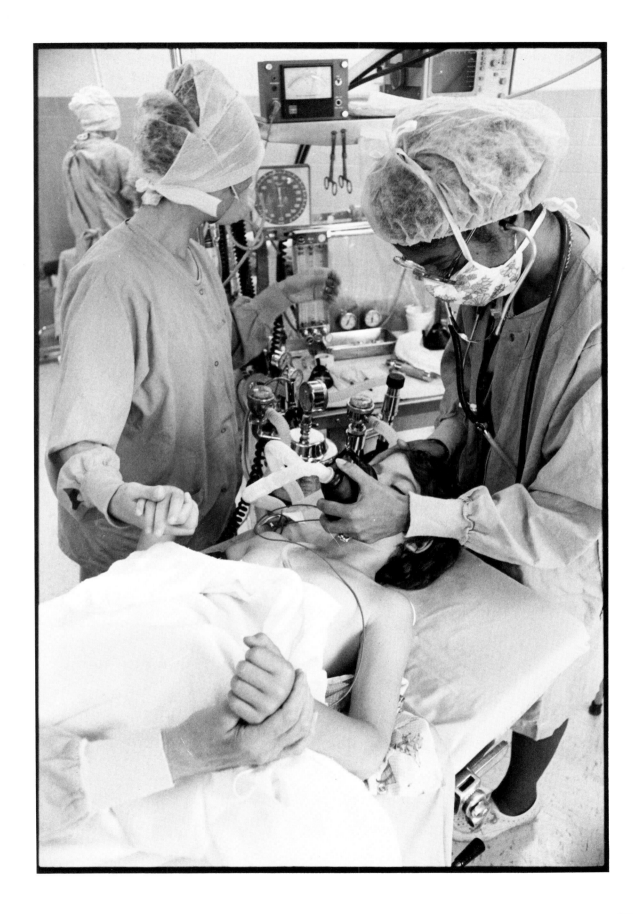

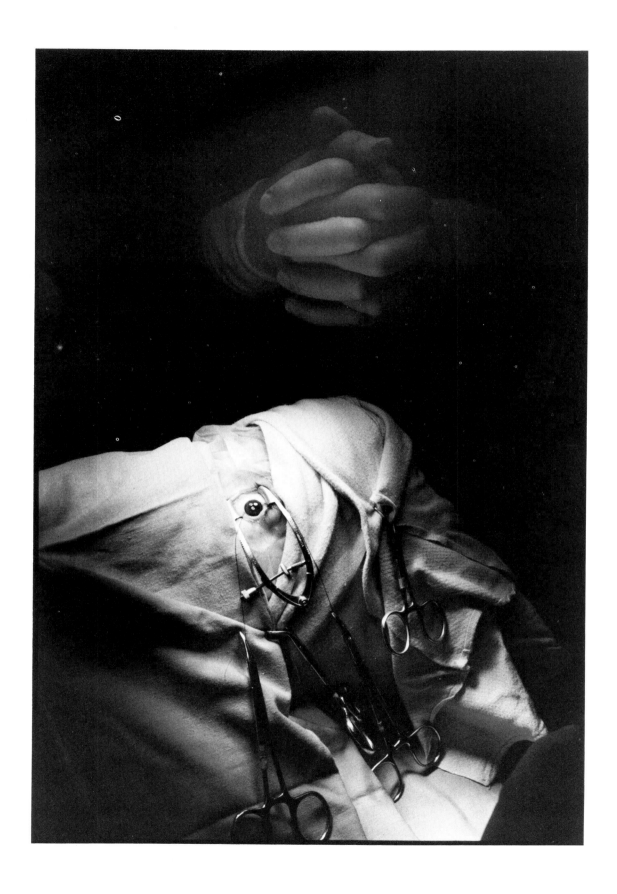

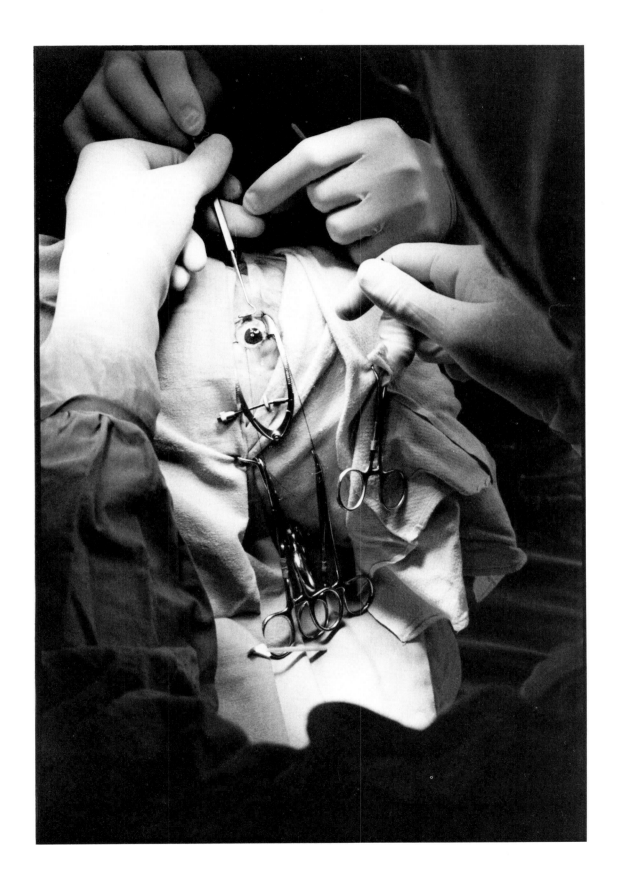

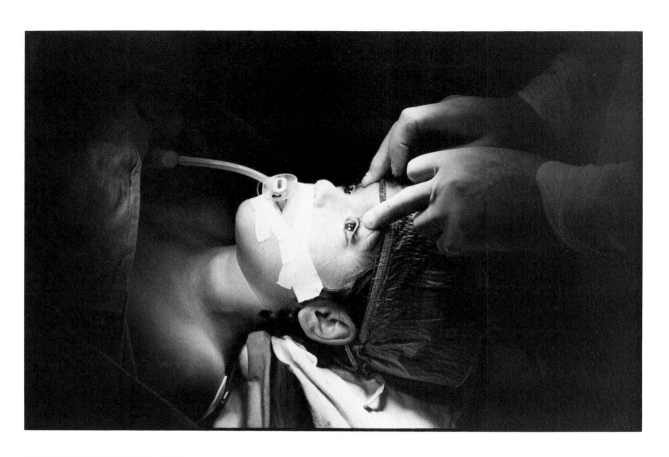

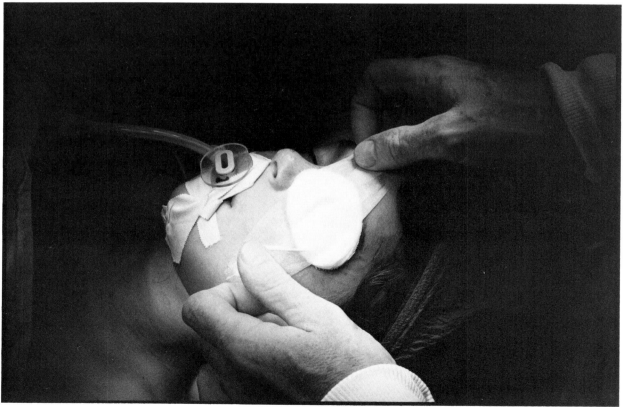

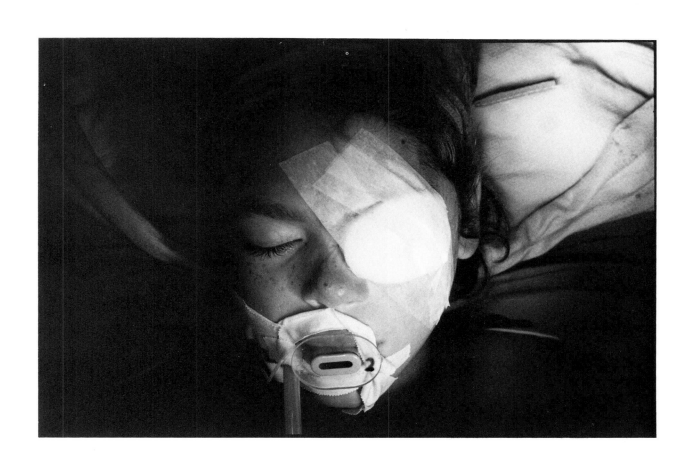

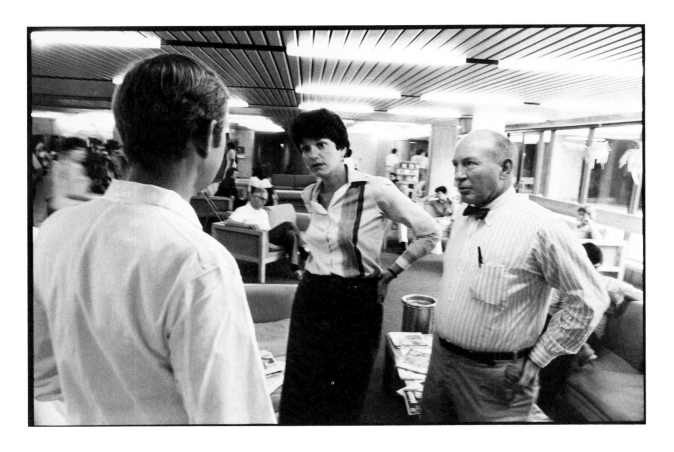

MRS. MONROE:

*I can't imagine what it would be like to wait with your child's life at stake. It's so traumatic. I don't know what I'd want—somebody to hold my hand the whole time, I guess. It's much harder to watch someone else go through it than to be the patient yourself. You just don't know what it's feeling like, what the pain is like, what her eye is going to be like, and how she's going to be when she comes back.*

July 16, 1979

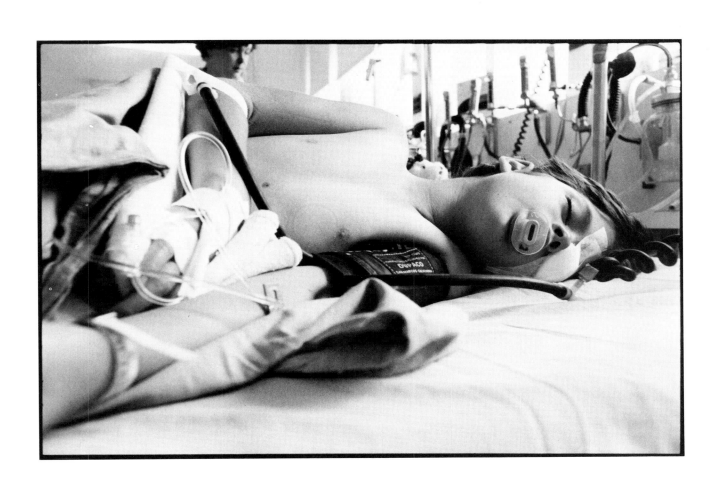

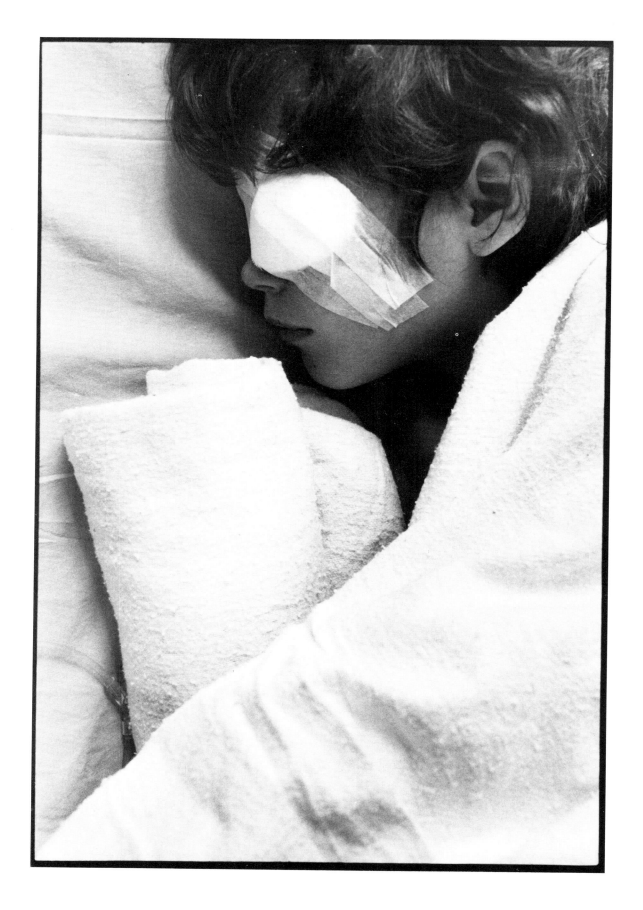

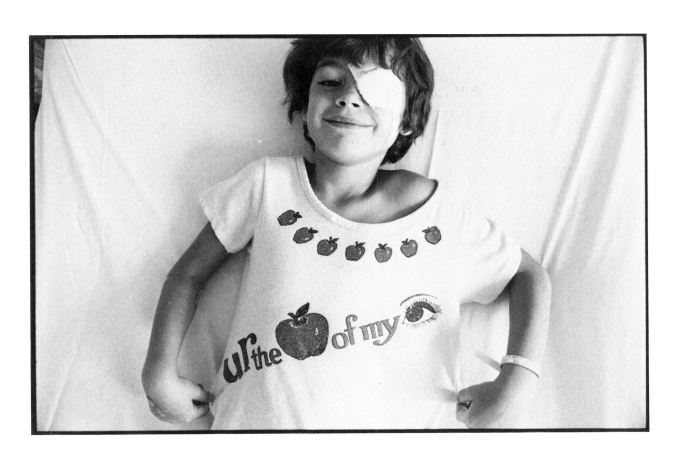

JENNY MONROE:
*I breathed and then I fell asleep, and then I found myself awake,*
*asleep in my room.*

July 17, 1979

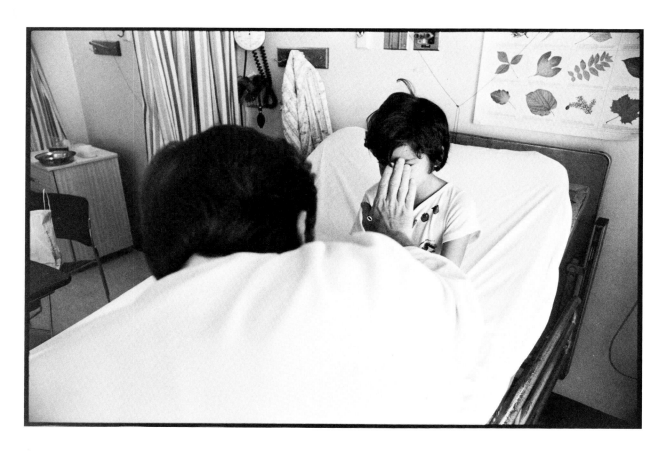

JENNY MONROE:
*He said, "O.K." and just tore the patch off and it hurt like mad*
*because I had stitches in my eye.*

July 21, 1979

MRS. MONROE:
*When Jenny woke up she was quite angry with me and grouchy.
She was in pain—like she had a piece of glass in her eye—and
she lashed out at me. I think she thought it was all my idea or
something. On the one hand I was relieved that she could
express her negative feelings and didn't feel she had to exhibit
perfect behavior; on the other I felt like I'd been here 3 days and
2 nights, sacrificed and done all this, why the hell was she
getting angry with me.*

July 17, 1979

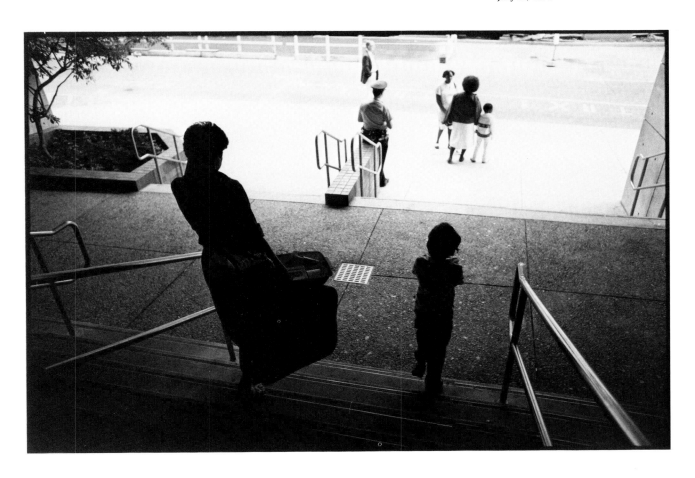

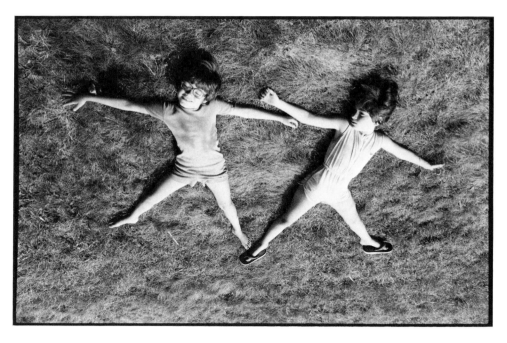

JENNY MONROE:
*Now I'm really embarrassed because my eye's all red and people are just going to be staring at me. I always see people whispering and I don't like that.*

July 21, 1979

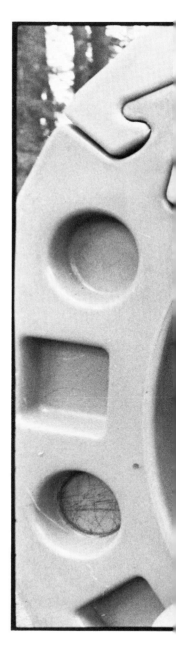

JENNY MONROE:
*I mean my sister just saw it yesterday and she goes, "Oh,
gross!"*

July 21, 1979

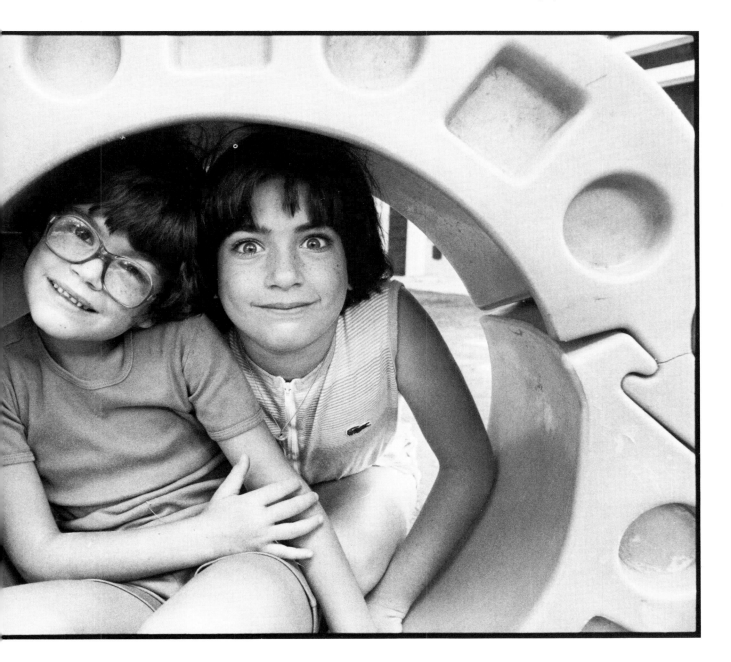

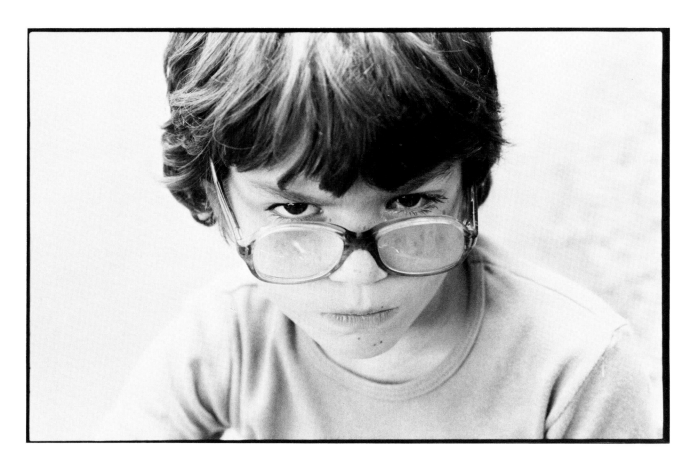

DR. MONROE:
*Shortly after the operation she had some behavioral problems; a lot of thumb-sucking, crying, and fighting with her sister. We didn't relate it to her eye—we just thought she was going through a phase. The question came whether Jenny had a poor body image: one doctor asked her if she liked herself, and Jenny wasn't sure.*

October 21, 1979

MRS. MONROE:
*But she never talked a lot about her eyes or how she felt about wearing glasses. I've seen that with a lot of things about Jenny.*

October 21, 1979

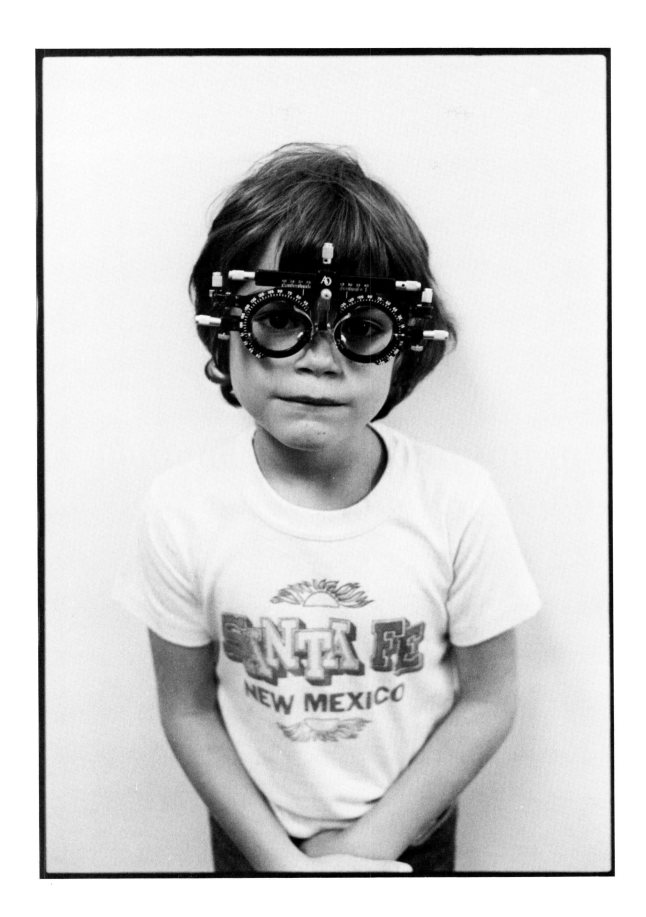

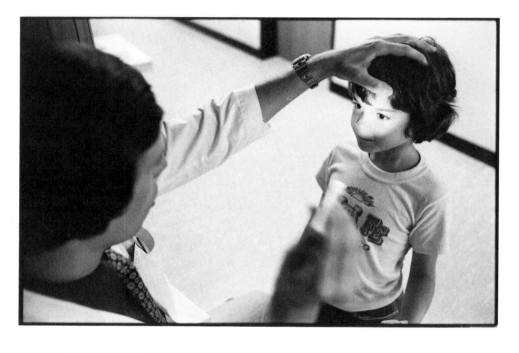

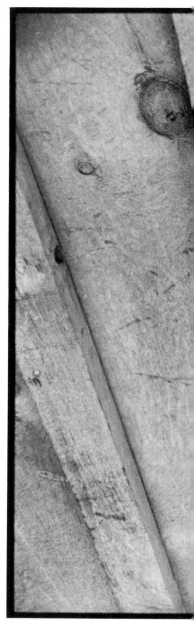

MRS. MONROE:

*I guess I had always underrated the significance of Jenny's wearing glasses—we hadn't thought that some of Jenny's behavior this summer could have been due to her problems with the glasses and the operation. But her physician noticed that Jenny focused on her eyes, and felt badly about them.*

October 21, 1979

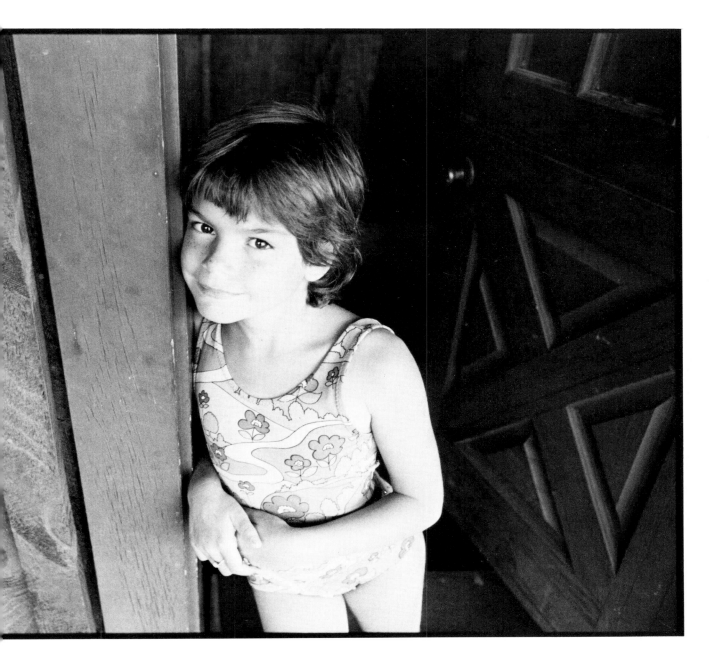

MRS. MONROE:
*I think she feels better about herself now. She's a little more confident, and seems to be happier at school...maybe—but just maybe—that has something to do with her eye.*

October 21, 1979

# Sandra Heywood

Sandra Heywood was 20 years old in 1970, when she developed signs and symptoms of rapidly worsening kidney disease. The precise cause of her disease could not be determined. Shortly after her condition was diagnosed, she underwent an operation to remove both her kidneys. During the next month, she spent six to eight hours a day, three days a week, in the hospital attached to a dialysis machine which removed from her blood the impurities and waste products normally removed by the kidneys. After discharge from the hospital, she continued to undergo regular outpatient dialysis treatments three times a week.

Two months after her first surgery Sandy received a kidney transplant but the transplanted kidney had to be removed because her body rejected it. Complications from the transplant and her kidney disease forced Sandy to spend the next sixteen months in the hospital. One of these complications was a progressive bone disease which, in 1975, led to two more operations in which parts of both hips were replaced with artificial joints. Sandy was in a wheelchair and then on crutches for almost two years after that.

Sandy returned to school in 1976, received her high school equivalency certificate two years later, and then enrolled as a part-time university student. As of November 1979, she was still receiving regular outpatient dialysis treatments while pursuing a degree as a medical technologist.

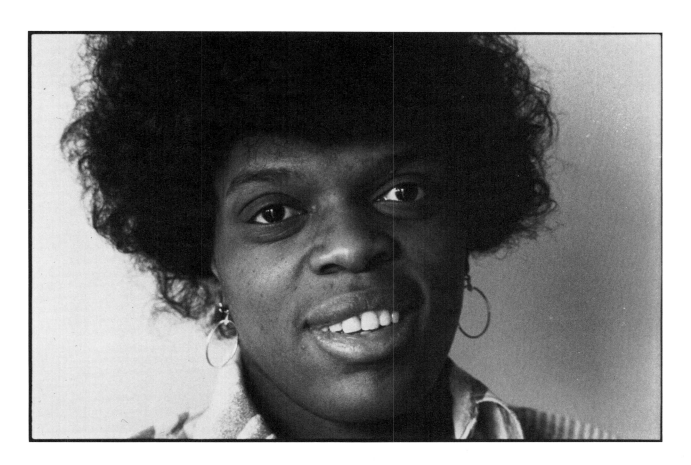

SANDY HEYWOOD:

*I didn't see any sense in just staying put, so I had dropped out of school and was driving a cab. It was my way of saying I could do what I wanted to do.*

*Then, one time I began to notice that my legs and hands were always swollen. I was really short of breath, and I was itching an awful lot. At the hospital they gave me an allergy test and they told me I was allergic to everything.*

November 22, 1976

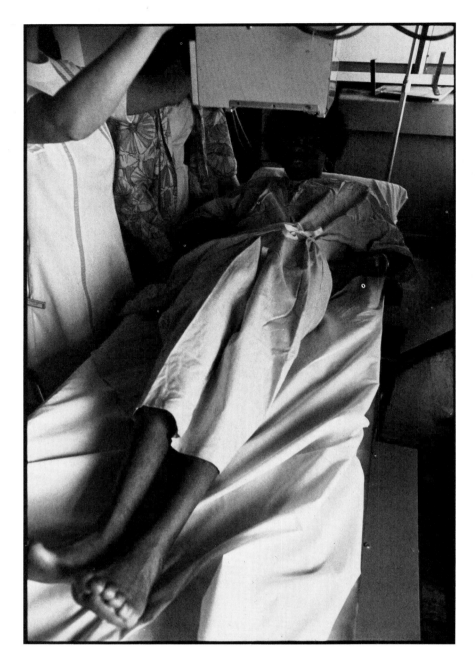

SANDY HEYWOOD:
*I was sitting there in the doctor's office chewing aspirins, when the doctor happened to ask me what I was chewing on. I used to get these real severe headaches from high blood pressure so I had started off with a small pack of aspirins and the next thing I knew I was on a whole bottle a day. I told the doctor and oh, my nerves, he almost had a fit. He ordered X-rays of my kidneys and that's how they found out my kidneys were failing. Nobody else in my family had ever had kidney disease so the doctor said something in the aspirins had probably made my kidneys fail.*

December 22, 1976

SANDY HEYWOOD:

*When they told me they had to take my kidneys out I just said it couldn't be possible. I had always been a healthy person and I hadn't even been in a hospital! I thought, "Why me?" I wondered if I were the cause of my own illness or if someone else had somehow caused it. Afterwards I found out that my illness is not hereditary and not my fault. It's God's nature, just something that happened.*

*They operated on me in January 1971 and took out both my kidneys. I had to stay in intensive care for two months.*

December 22, 1976

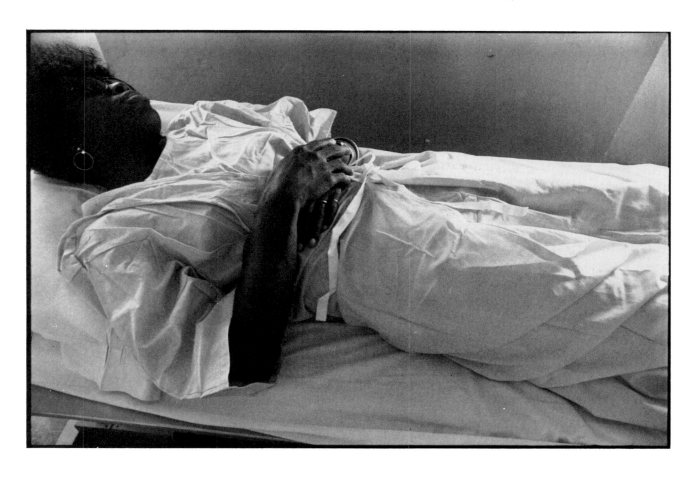

SANDY HEYWOOD:

*The first time I saw the kidney machine I thought it looked like a big washing machine. I said, "I hope you all aren't going to put me in that machine!" One of the nurses just started laughing and then she told me that they hook you up by needles. I didn't know anything.*

December 22, 1976

SANDY HEYWOOD:

*I was just twenty years old when I got sick and I could not accept being on dialysis. For a while every chance I got I tried to escape, and a few times I left the hospital still in my pajamas with my hospital band on. Sometimes they had to strap me down to the machine because I pulled those tubes out of my arms.*

*People have told me that when I escaped, threw tantrums, or tried not to show up for dialysis, that was my way of saying how I felt.*

December 22, 1976

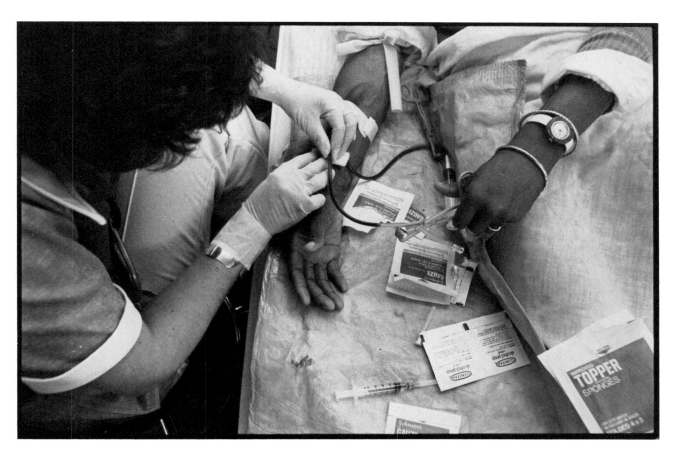

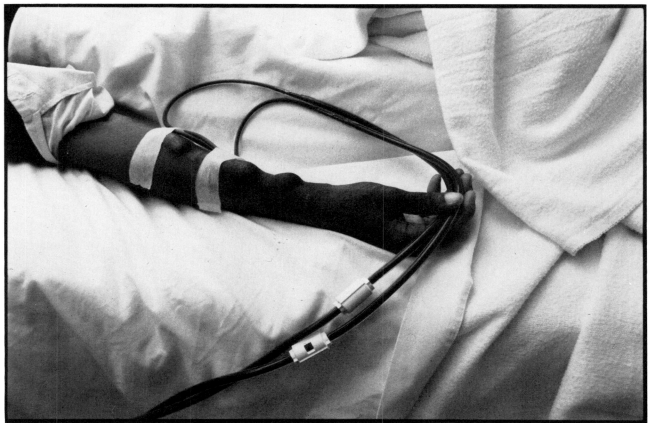

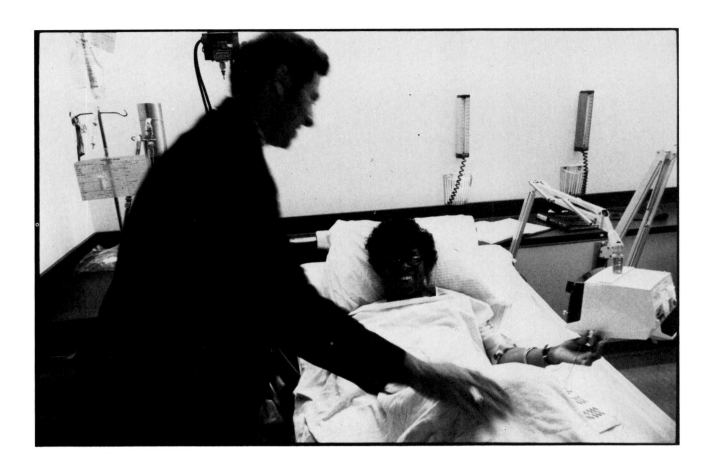

SANDY HEYWOOD:
*When I first got sick I didn't talk to the doctors and nurses
because I didn't know what they were talking about. They confused me and they scared me. It would have helped if they had
talked to me about everyday things.*

November 21, 1977

SANDY HEYWOOD:

*Two months after they took my kidneys out I received a kidney transplant. When I started having signs of rejection they had to take that kidney out too. It was kind of scary because I had a very high fever and lost my eyesight for twenty-four hours. A couple of times they didn't think I was going to make it because my temperature just wouldn't go down.*

December 22, 1976

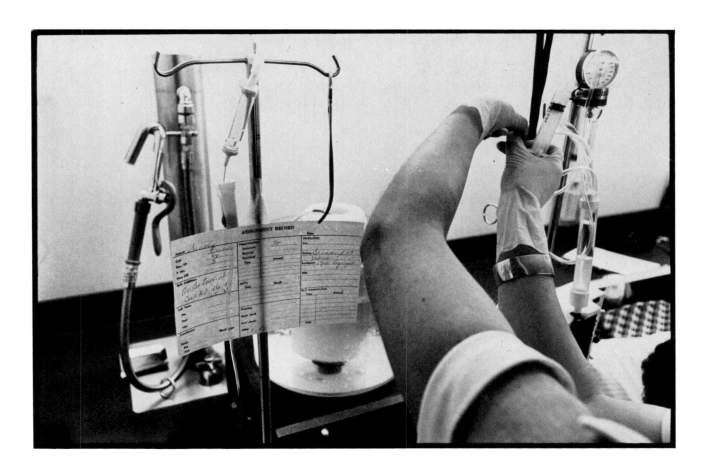

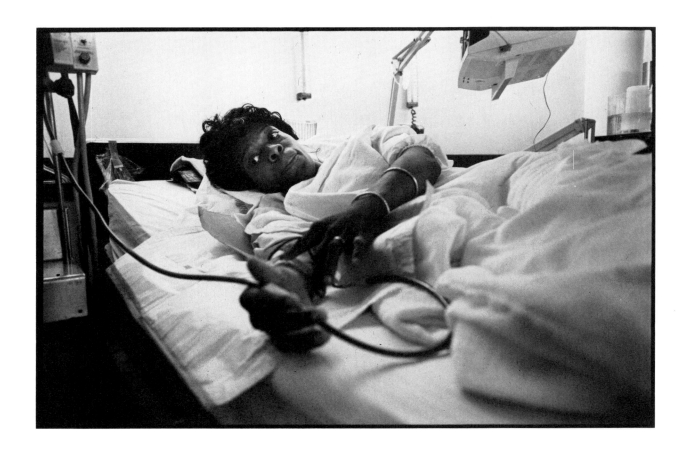

SANDY HEYWOOD:
*My father had a particularly hard time accepting my illness.*
*Any time he came to the hospital he would break out crying or*
*have to leave the room. He thought that I was going to be hooked*
*up to the machine for the rest of my life and that I could never*
*come home. That frightened him. He wanted to give me one of*
*his kidneys for a transplant, but his tissues didn't match mine.*
*When they told him that, he asked if he could take my place on*
*the machine. He didn't understand enough about dialysis to*
*know that I have to sit there because I have the kidney disease.*

December 22, 1976

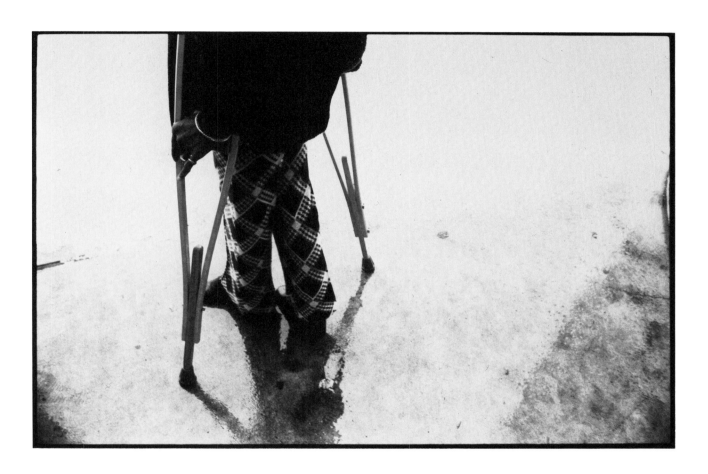

SANDY HEYWOOD:
*There were times when I was in a lot of pain and I didn't want to see anybody. I didn't really give a damn.*

*When I left the hospital, I was just exhausted. I couldn't even go out and shop for myself. People called to ask if I wanted to go out with them and I always had to say no. I was so miserable I figured that I would make them miserable.*

March 27, 1977

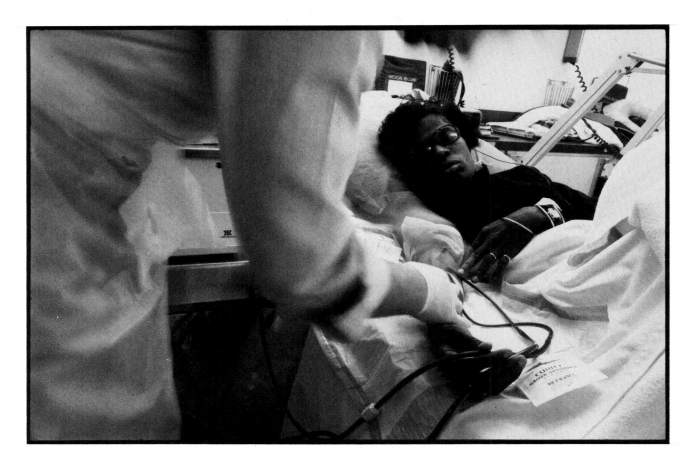

SANDY HEYWOOD:
*I had to go on a really crazy diet. For a while all I could eat was
a half bowl of jello. I could only drink so much of this and so
much of that, and I had to measure everything out, right to the T.
It was like hell to me. I was always hungry. I figured I could kick
the kidney problem if I didn't die of malnutrition.*

*One day I overdid it at dinner and I ended up back in the
hospital for a couple of weeks. It just didn't seem like anything
was going to go right.*

December 22, 1976

SANDY HEYWOOD:
*I had the urge to go to the bathroom, but every time I went
nothing came out. I began to think I was some kind of freak.
Finally I asked the doctor how come I wasn't going to the
bathroom and he said, "Didn't anybody tell you that when your
kidneys are out you don't urinate?" That was another crushing
blow because you take it for granted that you are going to wake
up in the morning and automatically have to go to the bathroom.
So after a while I just went to the bathroom and said what the
heck, I'll make believe I'm going.*

December 22, 1976

56

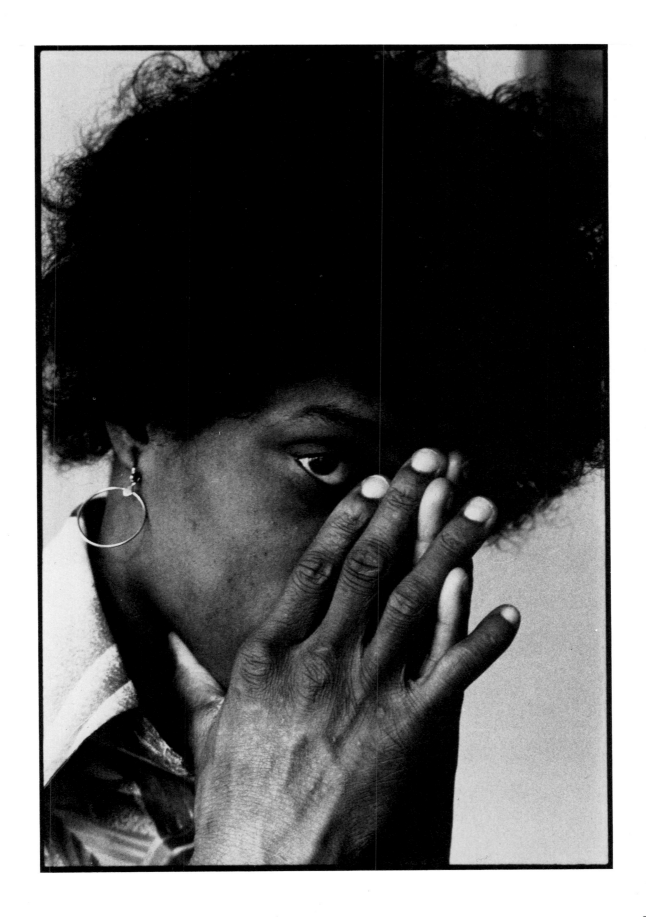

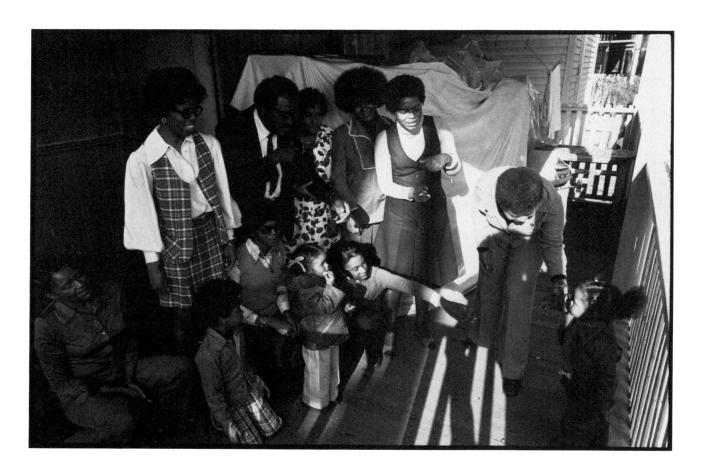

SANDY HEYWOOD:

My family and friends didn't really believe I had kidney disease. They took the same attitude I had taken at first. They just didn't want to see it. When I tried to talk to them about it, they thought I was crazy. Just because I look well on the outside doesn't mean I'm well on the inside.

One weekend we drove from Boston to New York. After everyone else had had to stop to go to the bathroom they said, "Damn, aren't you ever going to go to the bathroom?" I was too embarrassed to explain anything. But when I came back my doctor had a talk with my family. He told my family what to expect from somebody who had kidney failure. When I found out he had talked to them it wasn't so hard for me to talk.

November 21, 1977

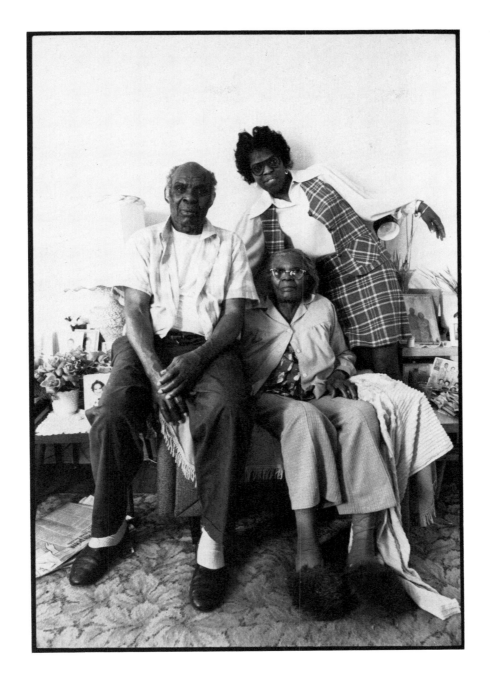

LAMBERT MOORE:
(Sandy's Grandfather)

*Sandy is very contented with her sickness. I see there's a lot of
people get sick and get disagreeable. They want to commit
suicide. But Sandy knows something about the grace of God, and
I think that's why she's holding out so good. I don't know how
long she can hold out, but as long as she can take it, it's all right
with me. Ought to be all right with her, too.*

March 27, 1977

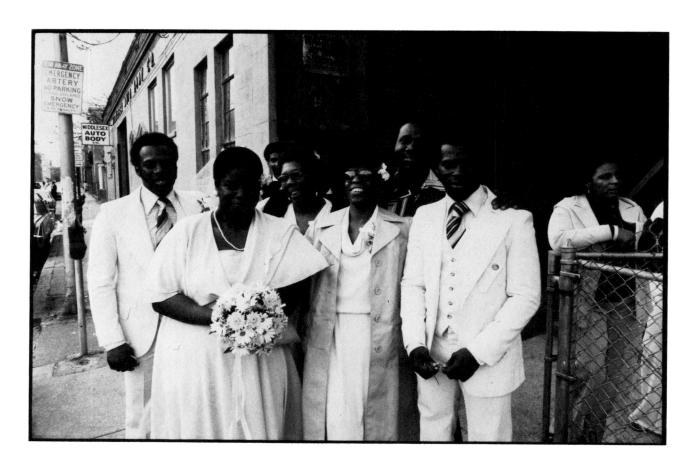

ELLEN LEVINSON:
(Social worker)
Sandy's family kept patting her on the back saying, "You've
made such a good adjustment." She felt that they viewed her as
super-human and she had to live up to that. She couldn't
complain, she couldn't ask for much.

January 24, 1977

ELLEN LEVINSON:

*Life on dialysis is full of restrictions: the diet is restricted, vacations are restricted, one's daily schedule is restricted. Everything has to be set up ahead of time. There's very little spontaneity left, everything has to be planned. On the other hand, dialysis hasn't been in existence long enough for anybody to know how long people who depend on it might expect to live. So patients are forced to plan their life without knowing how long it will be.*

January 24, 1977

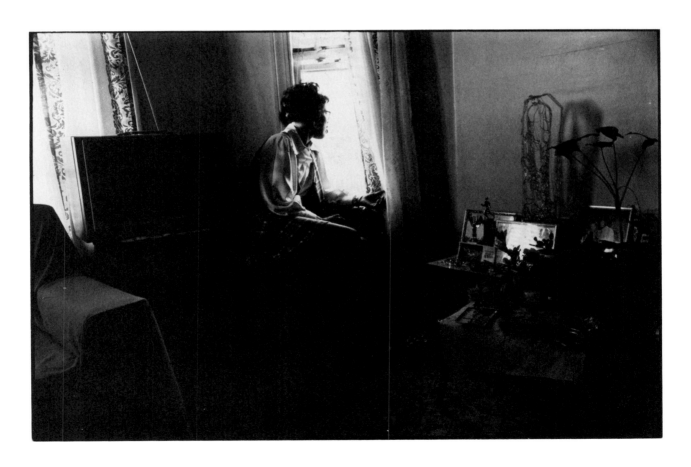

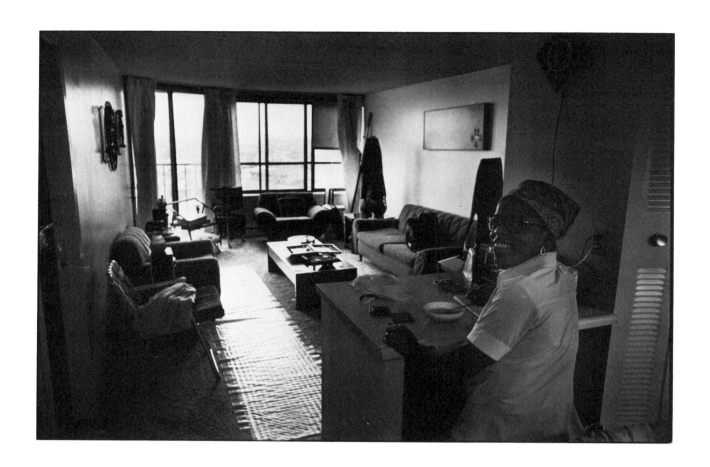

SANDY HEYWOOD:
*They asked me if I wanted to have dialysis at home, with my own machine in my own apartment. I told them there was no way that I wanted that there facing me all the time, always reminding me. I know that I have to go in for dialysis and that it has to be part of my life. But, damn, I won't let it run me.*

November 21, 1978

SANDY HEYWOOD:

*I have always been independent. When I first got sick, my mother wanted me to sell my car and live with her. She wanted to take what little independence I had away from me. Had she done that I would have been in trouble now. I would have sat around the house thinking about my kidneys all the time and crying the blues. Shoot, I wanted to go out and have fun.*

January 24, 1979

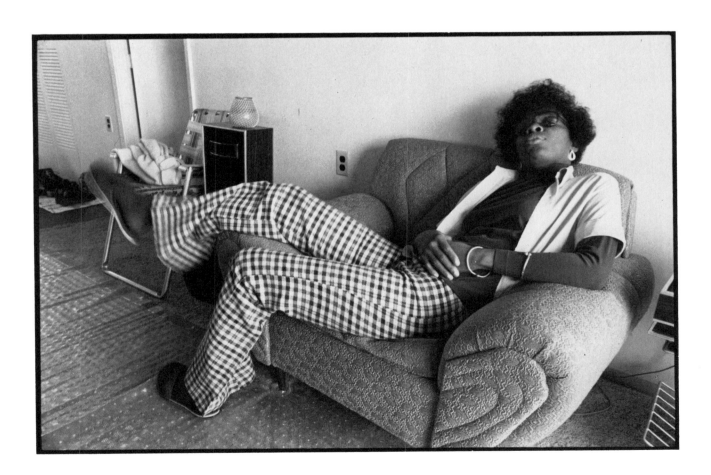

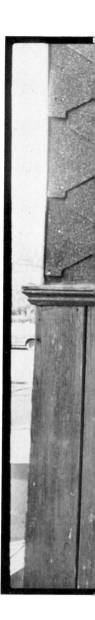

SANDY HEYWOOD:

*I don't feel sick like I did in the beginning. When I get out of bed now I don't feel like I'm going to fall over. I don't have so many headaches and I'm not as tired as I used to be. I go out and do most of the things I did before I got sick. The more I get out, the better I feel.*

March 27, 1977

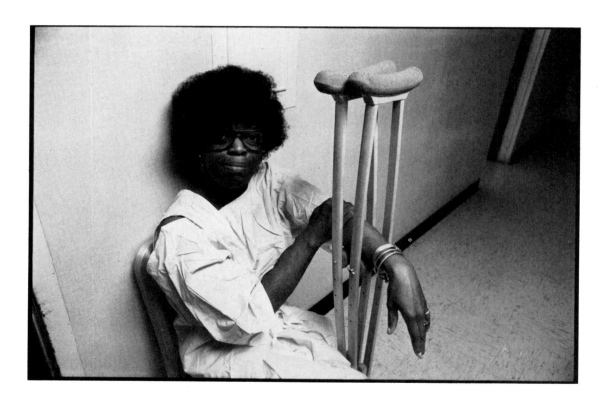

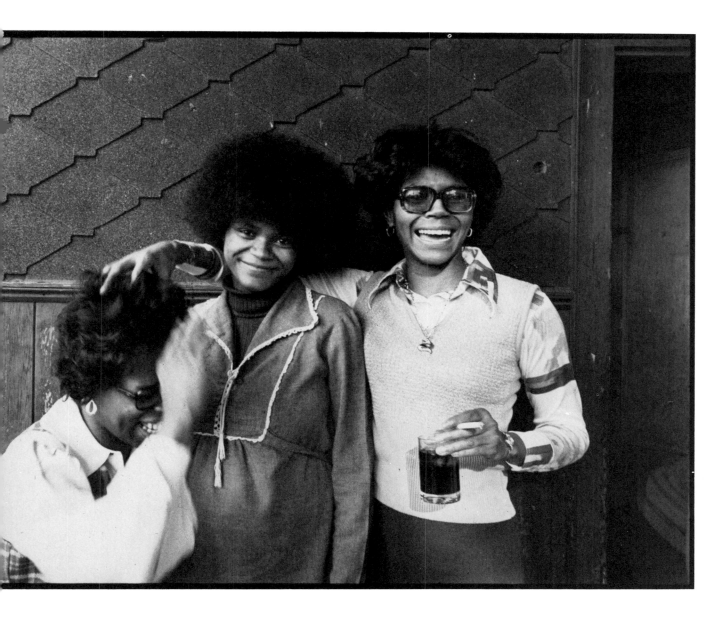

SANDY HEYWOOD:
*My cousin doesn't treat me special because I have kidney problems. We still go out and shop, or go to a party and have a good time, without her reminding me, "Don't do this," or "Don't drink too much because you're not supposed to." You know, it's not necessary.*

March 27, 1977

SANDY HEYWOOD:

*A lot of people told me I was crazy to get a moped, that it was too dangerous. I guess they thought that because of my condition I should sit around and twiddle my fingers. But my medical doctor told me it would probably be good for me, good for my spirits.*

November 27, 1977

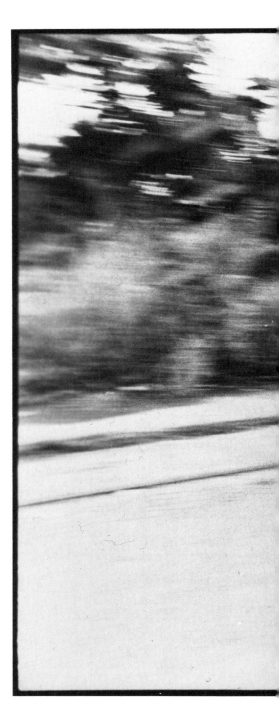

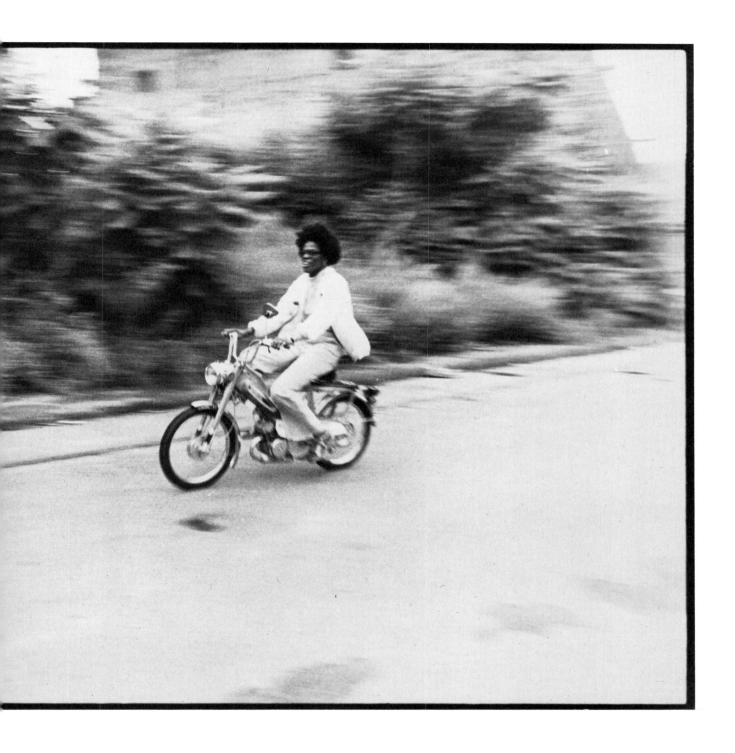

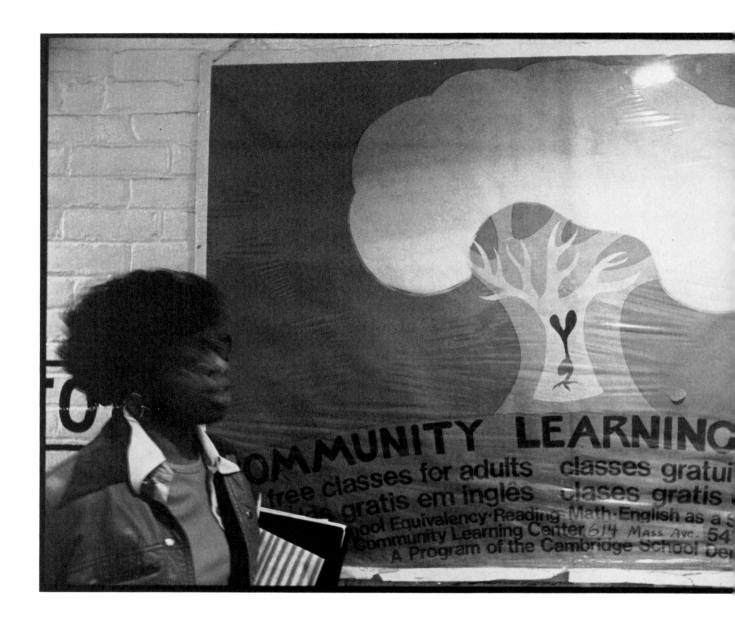

SANDY HEYWOOD:
*When I was first applying to school they didn't want to accept me. I guess they thought I was going to have a heart attack or croak on them. A lot of people, when they hear I'm on dialysis, expect me to be half-dead.*

March 24, 1977

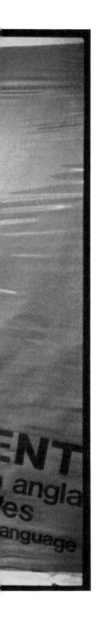

Graduation Speech—Excerpts from Valedictory Address
June 20, 1977

*If opportunity knocked only once, I wouldn't be here tonight. Dropping out of school was a mistake, and graduating this time wasn't easy. There were times when the problems caused by my illness seemed too much for me. But, then, I got tired of being depressed and sick. I came to realize that the value of my experience was* something else!

*I am now planning on going to college to obtain a degree as a medical lab technician. I hope to be able to give doctors and other people a different perspective on the diseases they study.*

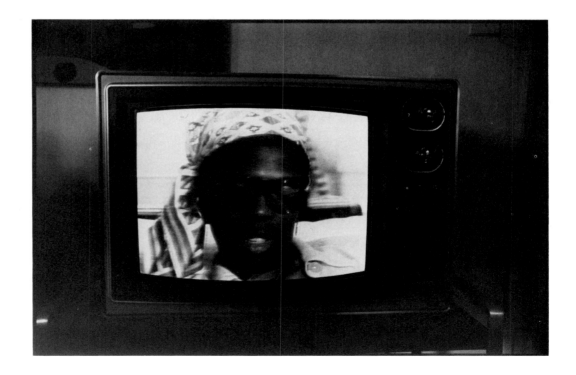

SANDY HEYWOOD:

*I had a chance to put my schooling to use recently. I was offered a job that pays $10,000. But the same system that pays all this money for my education and rehabilitation puts too many obstacles in front of me.*

*If I had taken the job, Medicare and Medicaid would have stopped paying for my medical expenses which amount to about $2000 a month. So I had to refuse it.*

*I'd like to get paid like anybody else. I'd like to have my own pocket change. I'd like to be able to afford a movie once a week.*

June 21, 1979

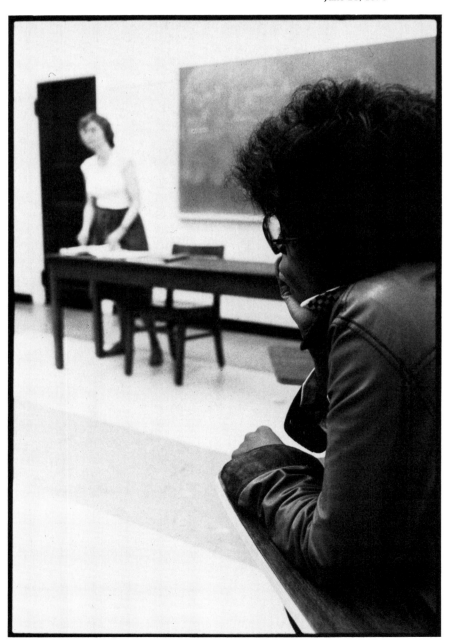

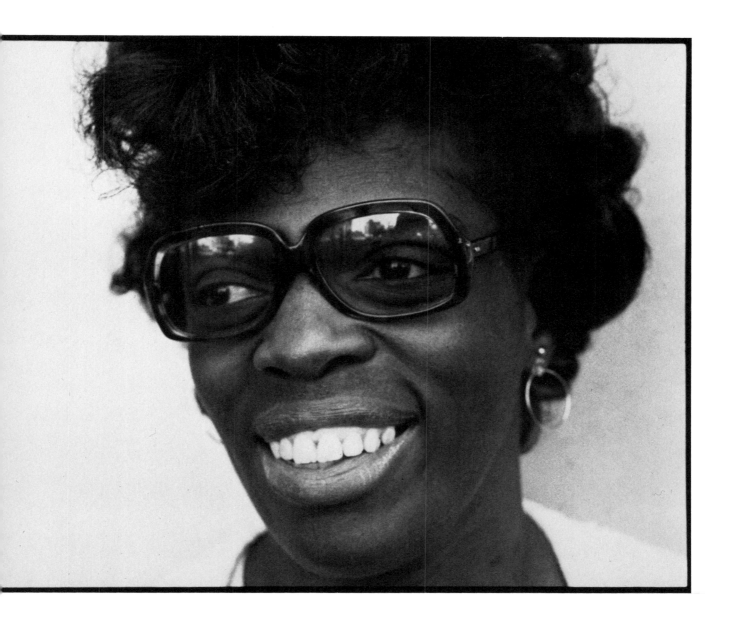

SANDY HEYWOOD:
*Enjoying life to the fullest would mean not having to worry about*
*being on dialysis and not having to go back and forth to doctors.*
*It could be better, but it's not really bad now.*

June 21, 1979

SANDY HEYWOOD:

*I figure I was on my deathbed twice, times when everybody taking care of me didn't think I was going to live. But as sick as I was I'm still here. When an article about me appeared in the paper recently, one of my doctors who had seen me at my worst stages said he was tickled pink at my accomplishments. I bet that in his mind he was thinking. "I didn't think she was going to make it. We might have pulled the plug..."*

November 21, 1978

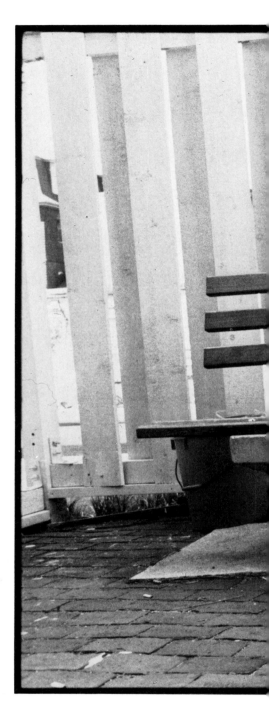

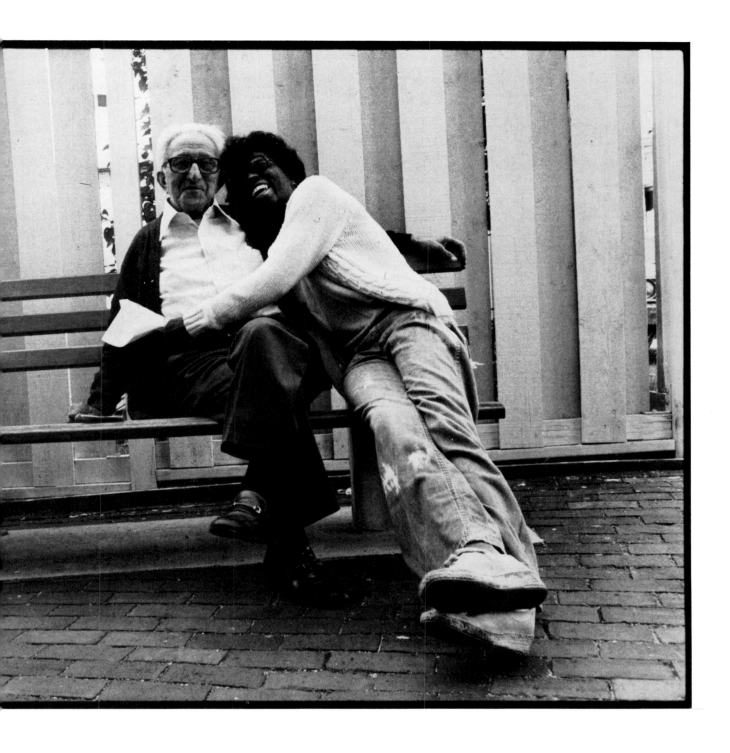

# Kathleen Finn

By the time Kay Finn first sought help for breast cancer in October 1976, she had been living with pain in her breast and back for more than a year. She was 63 years old and lived at home with her sister who was 70. The physicians who saw her in the tumor clinic thought her disease was too advanced for surgical treatment. She underwent a breast biopsy to give the physicians the information necessary to decide whether she could be treated effectively with hormones. She remained at home for another month before she was admitted to an acute-care hospital for three weeks. She was then transferred to a chronic-care facility, where she died in February 1977.

KAY FINN:

*It was getting too much for me. Really it was. The heaviness and everything else about it was getting too much for me. I knew I had to go and that was all there was to it. I had no choice.*

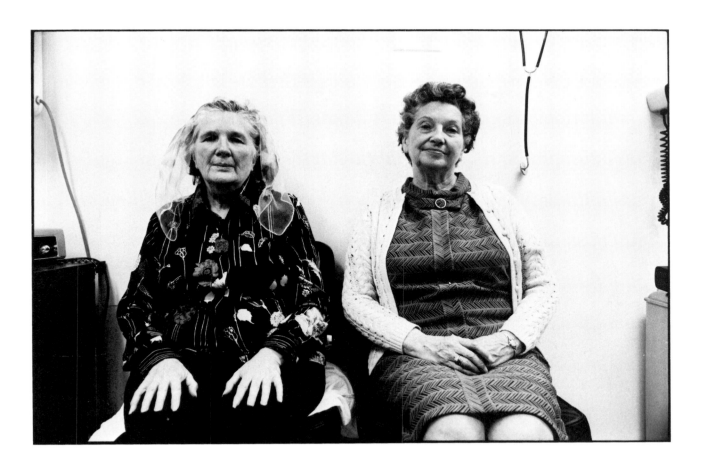

KAY FINN:

*I say to my kids, "Don't you worry, I will live to one hundred. My grandmother did." I know the doctors will pull me through. So I keep saying I will live, they will have to shoot me....*

*They never hear complaints. I just say let me get through this and I am going to enjoy my life.*

November 12, 1976

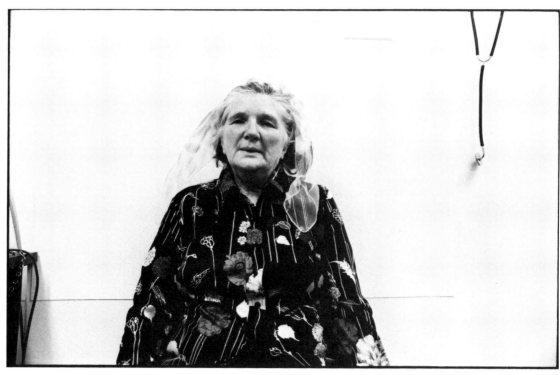

KAY FINN:

*I want to keep a cheerful attitude going through life because that is the only thing I ever had going for me. I avoid anyone that I feel is going to comfort me because I don't want them to get me down.*

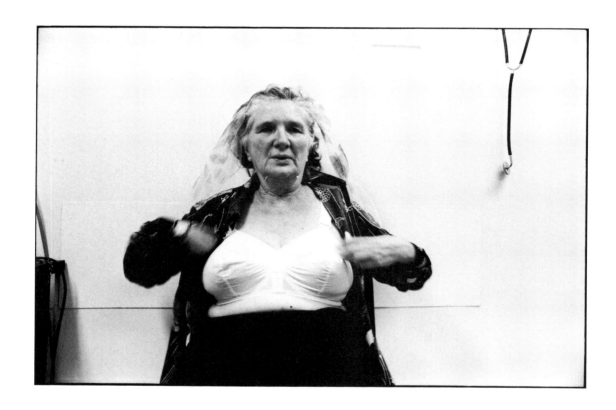

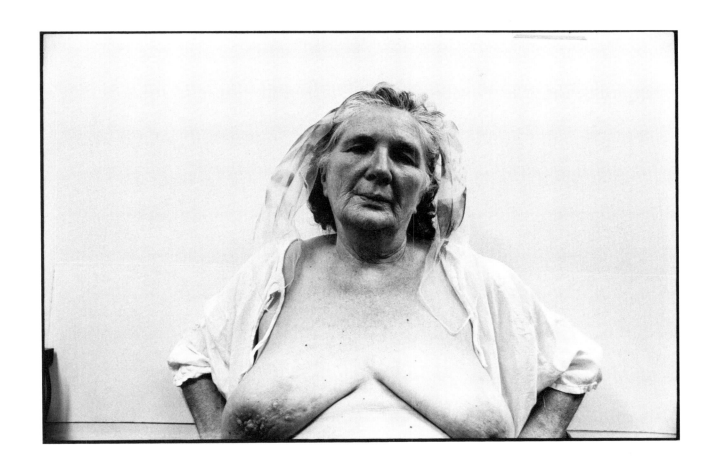

DR. FROMM:
(Surgeon)
*I interpreted her explanation of how she has helped other people with
her good spirits as saying, "Why should this happen to me?" I was
also struck by her absolute denial of what is going on.*

November 19, 1976

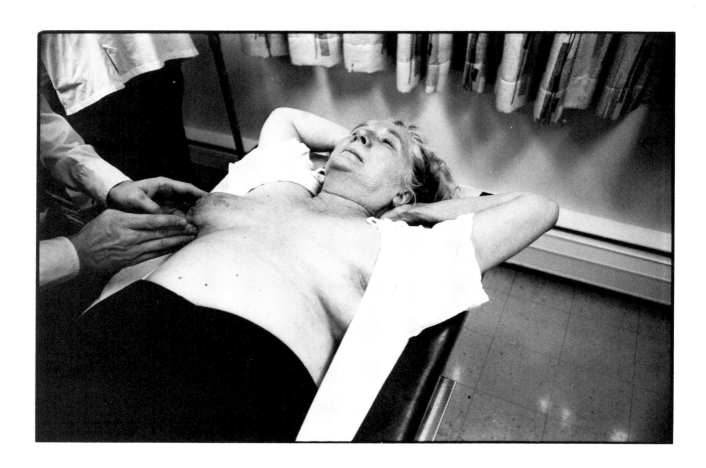

KAY FINN:

*He just examined me.*
*They all examined my breasts,*
*and they said it was massive tumors.*
*That's all.*

November 19, 1976

MARY McCARTHY:
(Mrs. Finn's sister)

*She told me she had said to the doctor, "What about, you know, operating on my breast?" And he said: "What about it?..." See, he didn't answer her. And they never operated on her breast. The doctor told me it had spread through her body and there was really nothing they could do. She just told me about it and that was it. She never said any more about it.*

November 19, 1976

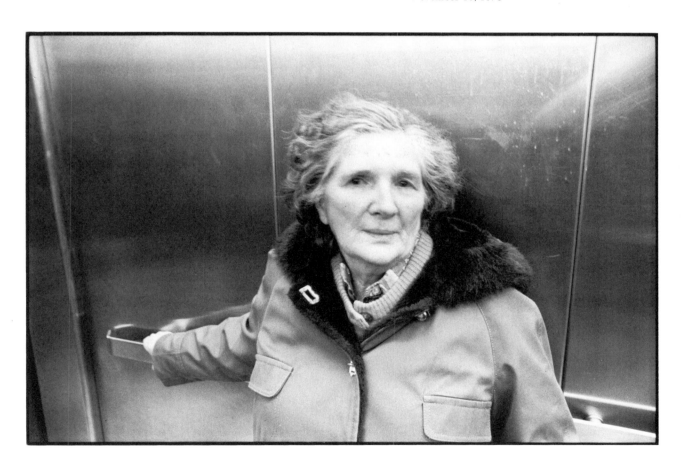

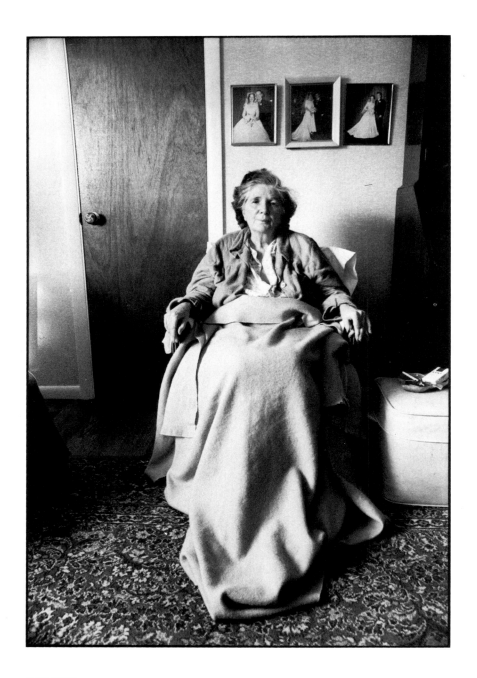

KAY FINN:
*I have nothing.*

*I lead what someone else would think is a very dull life. But I led that all my life, so that is nothing new. All I did in life was be married and work when I could. I didn't work in the second marriage for twelve years, but I was perfectly content to be at home.*

*And I still am that way.*

November 14, 1976

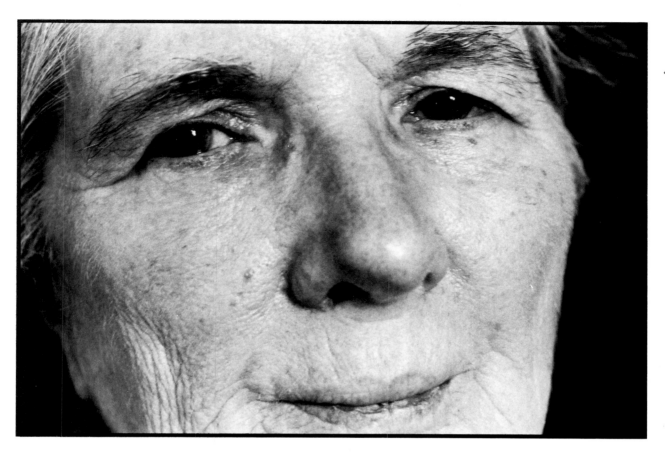

KAY FINN:
*I have a sense of humor and I want to keep it. I was never noted for being a cranky person and that is what I'm afraid of: the change in my personality. I don't want to be an irritable person, or a crank, or a pain. That's all.*

November 14, 1976

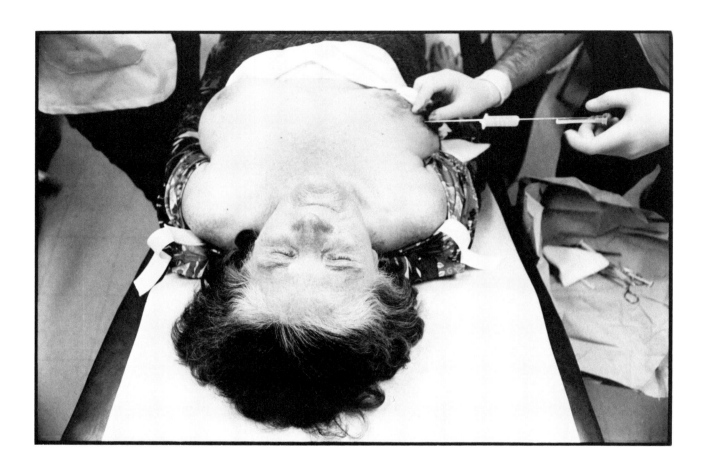

KAY FINN:
*I am a little afraid of it.*

*That is a hard thing, to be afraid of pills and afraid of radiation.*
*I don't want a dependency on pills for the rest of my life. Too many of*
*my age group need pills for this and that and the other thing. The only*
*thing that keeps them going is pills.*

November 19, 1976

MARY McCARTHY:

*She had been up all Sunday night with pain, so the next morning we came in by ambulance to the emergency ward. I didn't know what was happening because I had to sit outside. They were taking her for X-rays and different tests but I didn't know where she was. Finally, when Kay was brought back, the lady doctor told me, "We will get her up and walking." But she couldn't walk. And the doctor said she was in no more pain; but she still was. They were trying to kid me along, that's all. Maybe calm me down.*

November 27, 1976

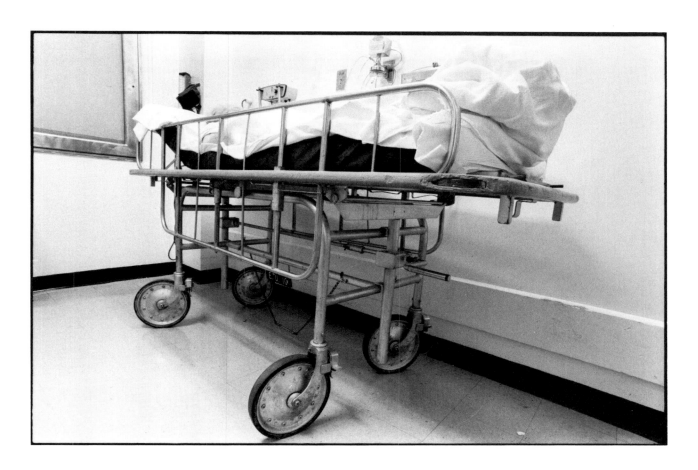

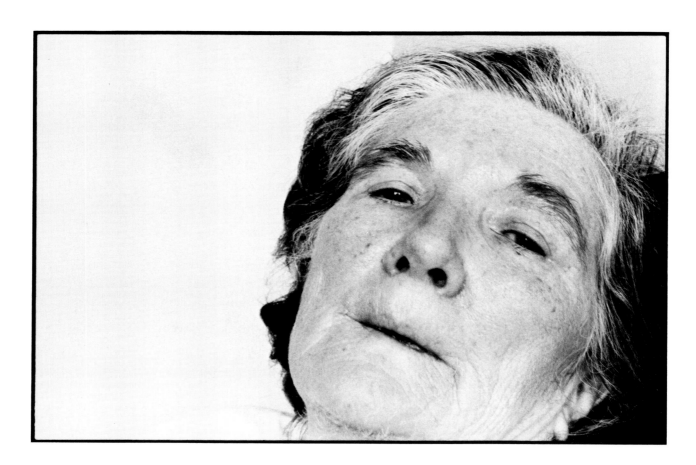

MARY McCARTHY:

*When we got home by ambulance we gave her the pills and made her as comfortable as we could. During the night I'd hear her in pain, and I'd run in, and she would say "it's just a pain." I watched and gave her the pills on time again.*

*Morning comes and she doesn't eat. The nurse told me to get that instant breakfast drink, and she does take that for me. She will never eat prunes but she ate a couple for me the other day. Since she won't eat steak for me, I figured that meat loaf is easier. She ate two teaspoons of that yesterday and she said that it was wonderful. And it wasn't.*

*So this morning she had instant breakfast drink again and that is about it.*

November 28, 1976

MRS. FINN: *Oh, God, I thought I could hit the roof. This is bad pain, it's sharp. And when I say, "Oh, ah..." Mary will say, "What's wrong?" I'll say, "It's the pain. That's what's wrong."*

MRS. McCARTHY: *I come in thinking that she wants something...*

MRS. FINN: *No, when I want you, when I call your name...*

MRS. McCARTHY: *That's when you want me?*

MRS. FINN: *Yeah, but I mean when I say, "Oh" or "Ah"...*

MRS. McCARTHY: *You don't want me then?*

MRS. FINN: *No. What the hell can you do about a pain that's inside your body?*

November 29, 1976

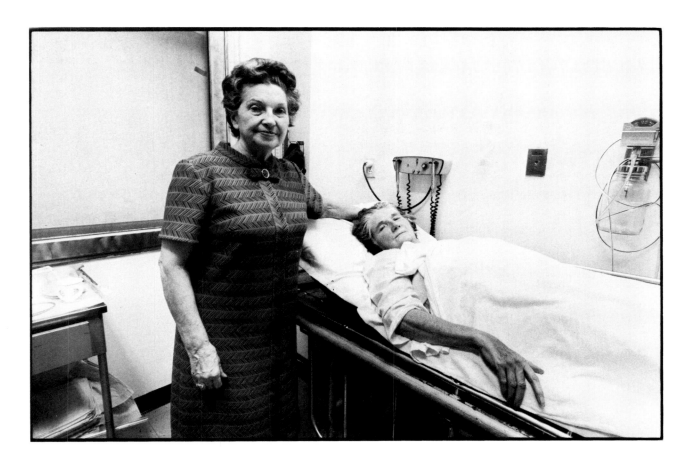

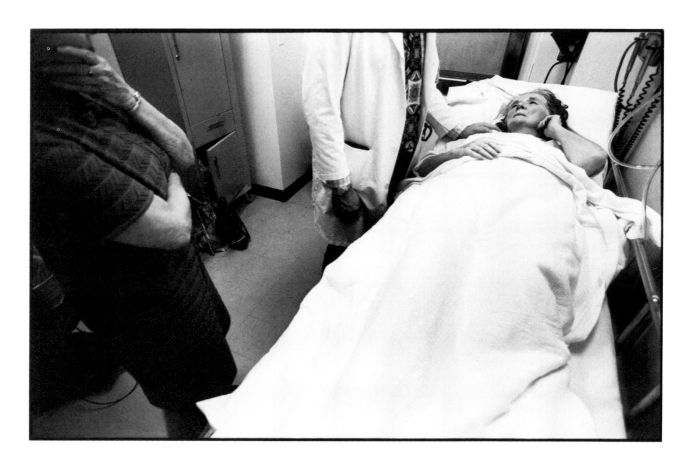

DR. LOWELL SCHNIPPER:
(Cancer Specialist)

*Mrs. Finn has been bedridden for about a week because of sudden, severe, and incapacitating back pain when she's standing. She has needed constant assistance at home. Her sister has difficulty dealing with this illness; she is terrified by the possible beginning of a terrible process, her impending death.*

*Her sister's son has really pleaded with me to take Mrs. Finn out of the home, not for her own sake, but because his mother is having a difficult time in helping her. He suggested that Mrs. Finn be placed in a chronic-care facility. But I am trying to avoid that just yet....She may not be ready to go into that continuous spiral leading to death.*

November 29, 1976

DR. SCHNIPPER:

*She has a very mournful appearance. She looks up with her sad eyes and asks that you help her, but she really doesn't indicate what kind of help she wants.*

*She looks as though she's been shattered, either by the news of the disease itself, or by understanding that in watching it for a very long time, she neglected herself and was probably instrumental in making herself a lot less treatable than if she had come to medical attention earlier. She felt ashamed that she hadn't taken care of it—probably because many of us asked her how long she had known she had a breast mass.*

*And I'm sure she's very, very frightened about what all this means to her now that she's permitted it to surface and become recognized...officially.*

November 30, 1976

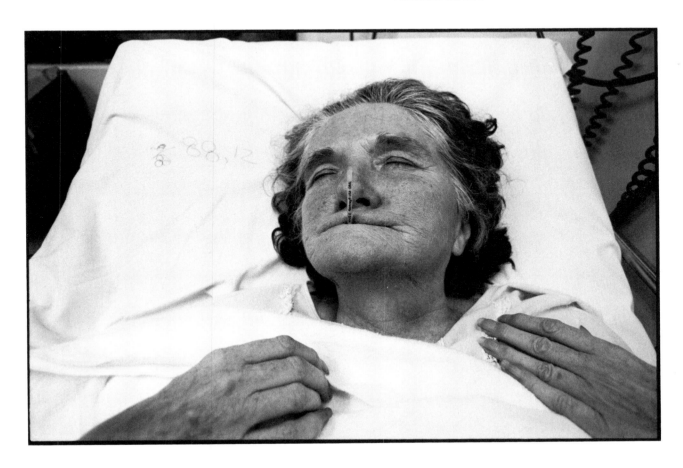

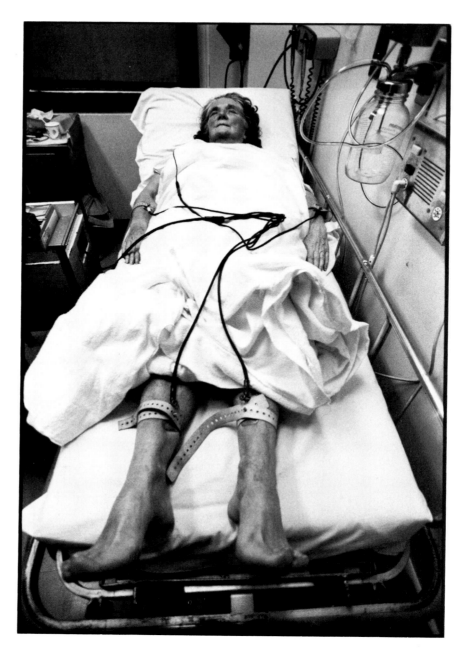

DR. SCHNIPPER:

*A major goal in our approach to patients with cancer is to keep them in the environment that they're most comfortable and familiar with...and not in the hospital, which, despite all our good intentions, is an alien and hostile environment to them.*

December 1, 1976

KAY FINN:

*They say why didn't I do something about it instead of letting it go like this.*

*After all, at sixty-three you're supposed to have brains enough to take care of yourself, brains enough to look into things and not be careless. They didn't come out with it like that, but I must look like a pretty careless person. I kept putting it off and putting it off, so I have no one to blame but myself actually.*

*I think I really and truly was looking for someone to come along with me, to give me moral support. I know I didn't want to go alone. For the first time in my life I was looking for someone to come along with me. I was looking for company badly, but I don't think the people I was talking to realized how badly I was wanting company. Because I tried to act so independent and underneath it all I'm not. I'm human, that's all.*

December 13, 1976

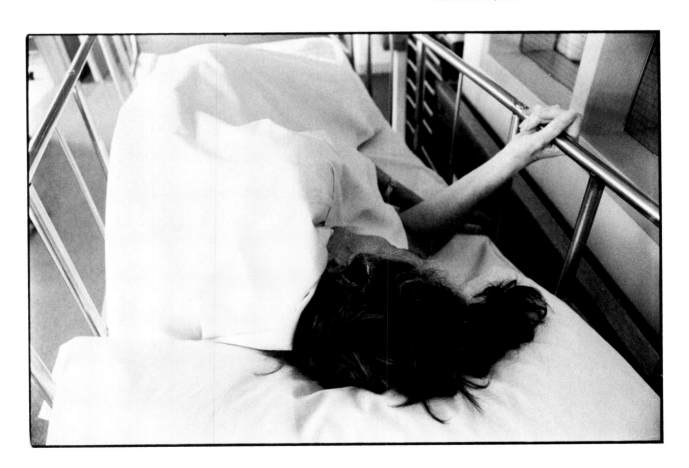

KAY FINN:

*I said how come the breast cancer goes down to the bones, why does that happen? And he says we don't know, but it does spread. Cancer does spread...I never realized that. I don't think that too many people anywheres realize that. So he says it's spread into the bones, that's that...*

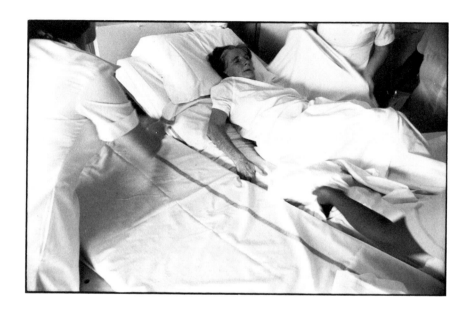

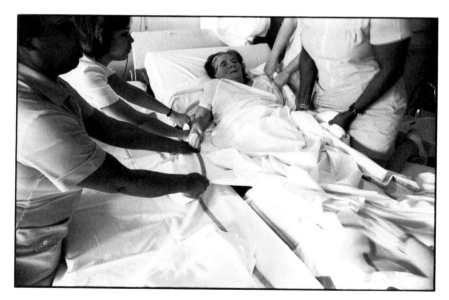

*...and as I say, when I can't straighten out...and I have to have two people help me...just a short distance...OOOOHH GOD...that's it...that's it.*

December 23, 1976

92

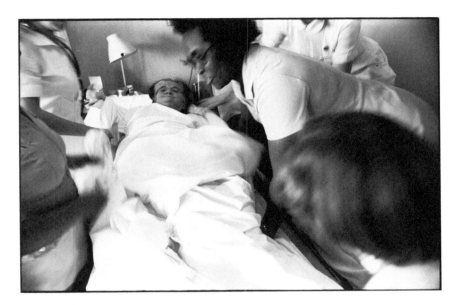

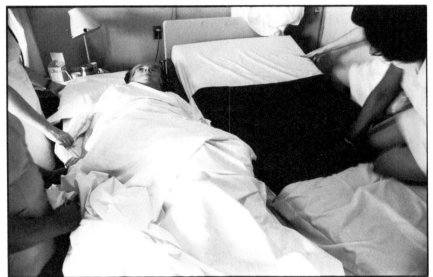

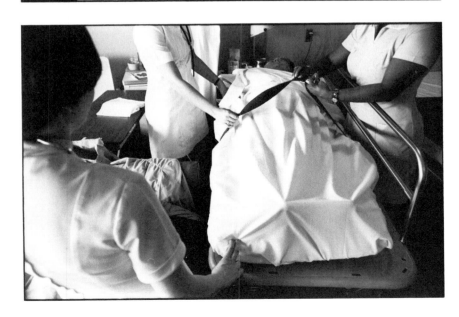

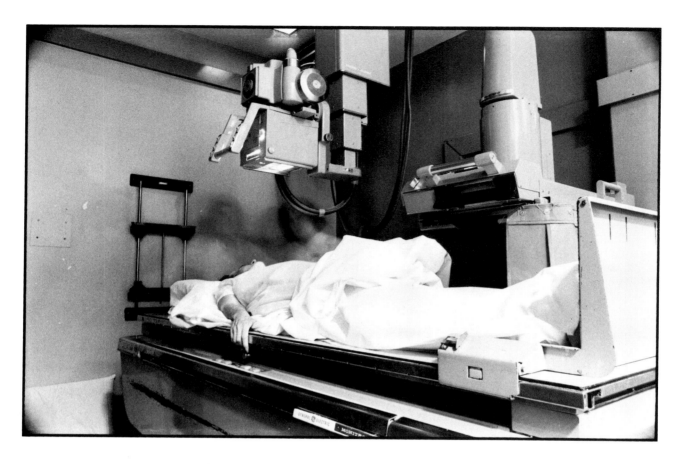

KAY FINN:
*It is getting up on the tables, that's when I feel things. It just hits me.*
*My back, oh God, it just hits me that I am in pain.*

MEDICAL RESIDENT:

*Well, here's an elderly lady with cancer of the breast and obvious metastases to the bone and presumably the liver and skull at this point. Needless to say, her prognosis is virtually nil at this point. She knows where she is but she has absolutely no insight into her situation at this point. In fact she is of the opinion that she'll be going home any day, and is incapable of realizing that she is not, despite repeated efforts by staff to tell her so. She essentially keeps repeating on and on that she wants to go home, and denies any particular concern about her impending demise...which I think is, quite frankly, beyond her understanding at this point.*

December 23, 1976

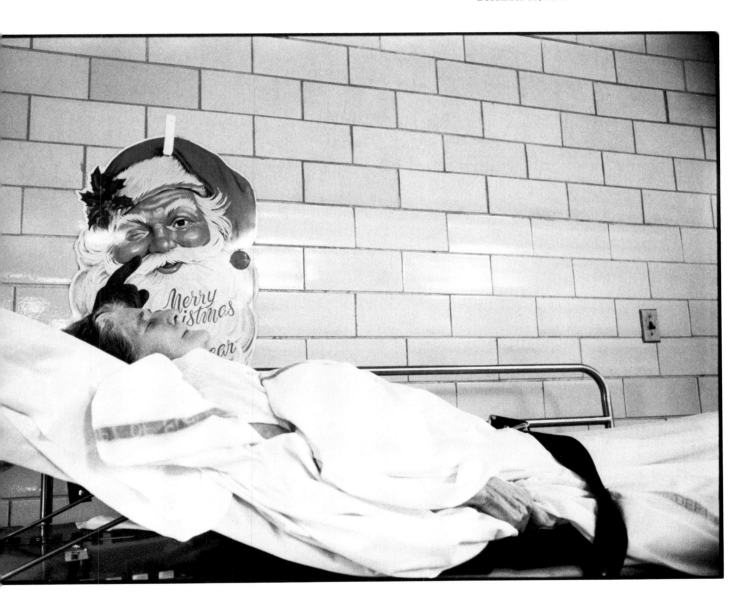

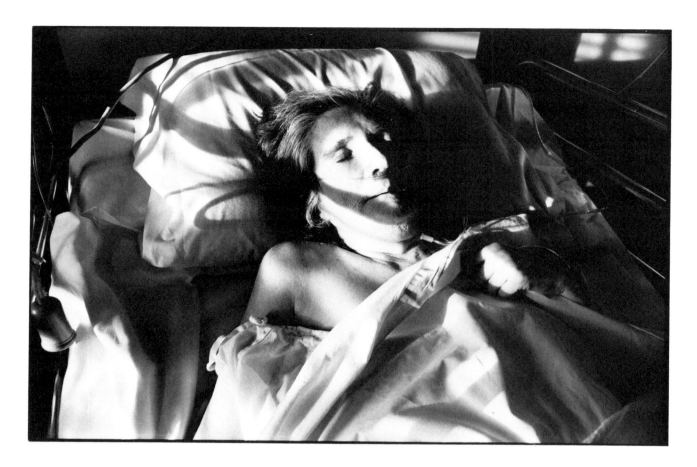

KAY FINN: *I'm afraid...I'm just petrified...Mary, I want you to stay. I'm afraid...I'm afraid of everybody...EVERYBODY!*

MARY McCARTHY: *I'll come tomorrow morning, Kay, right after Mass... all right?*

KAY FINN: *All right, but be careful 'cause I don't want no harm to come to you. Something could happen in five minutes.*

MARY McCARTHY: *Where?*

KAY FINN: *To this whole world.*

January 3, 1977

KAY FINN:
*If anything bothers me, stay away from me.*
*Leave me in peace.*
*That is it.*

January 8, 1977

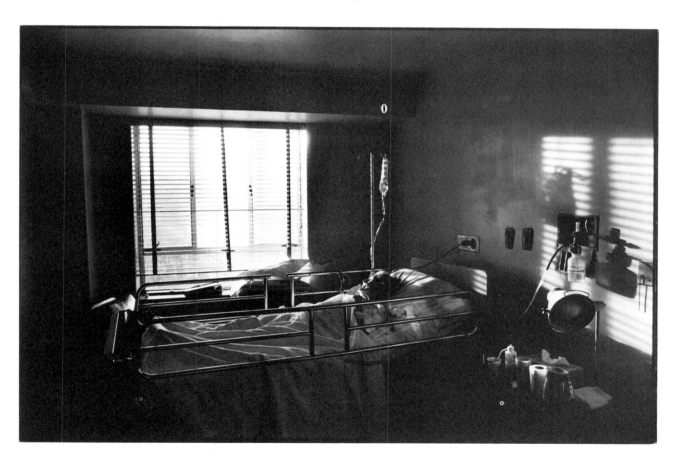

MRS. McCARTHY:

*People would say, "Oh, you shouldn't be goin' in every day." But I just had to see her. I felt that for my own peace of mind I had to see her. And she never complained. She was in that bed there and she was marvelous. She was really wonderful. She really was.*

*On February 3 Dr. Nicole called me and told me she had passed away. I was shocked, I was just shocked. I felt terrible to think that I hadn't gone in to see her that day...the one day I hadn't gone in.*

*But she was a person that didn't complain, that's the way she was. I think we're all like that in our family anyway.*

*I know once, here, before she had gone to the hospital, she said to me, "If anybody thinks I'm going to get better," she said, "they're whistlin' up a rope."*

March 3, 1977

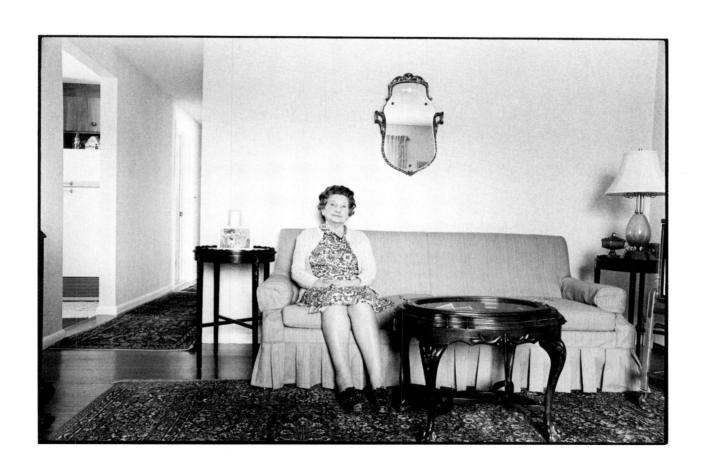

# Edwin MacPhee

Ed MacPhee was 53 when he underwent a coronary artery bypass graft operation in February 1979 for relief of severe and disabling chest pains. His chest pain, called angina, was due to blockages in his coronary arteries—the vessels that carry blood to the heart—which prevented his heart from receiving sufficient oxygen when stressed. The operation entailed removing a vein from his leg and using portions of that vessel to bypass the obstructed parts of his coronary arteries. His surgery and immediate post-operative course lasted 10 days and went well. Three days after his discharge, he was hospitalized at another hospital for psychiatric problems related to the stress of surgery.

Since his surgery he has had only mild and occasional angina and has significantly increased his level of activity. He was seen at a psychiatric outpatient clinic briefly until his psychiatrists felt this was no longer needed.

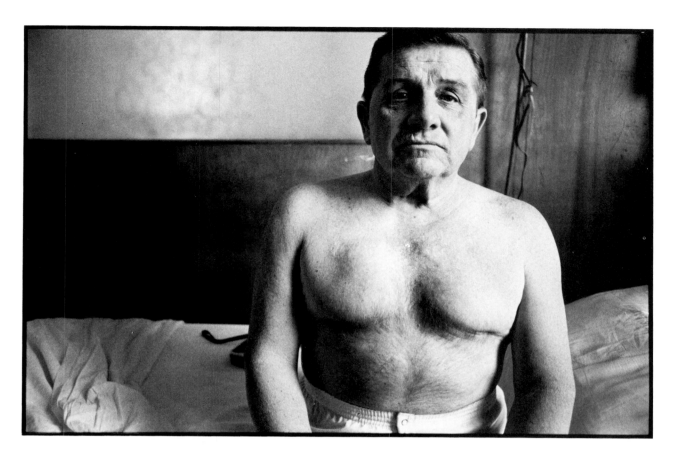

EDWIN MacPHEE:

*In 1963 I had this massive myocardial infarction. I was hospitalized for 30 days and I stayed home another 2 months recuperating. Eventually I regained my strength and was free to do everything. A certain portion of my heart had died, so I just slowed down and found that I could get along very nicely. No problem.*

*Then one day in 1976 I felt rather weak. I thought it was just the heat of the day, but I got off the train, sat down on the bench, and passed out. But I was so lucky, a police car took me to the Veterans Hospital where I passed out again. The cardiologist decided that I needed a pacemaker so I had a pacemaker installed in my right chest. I still have it to this day.*

January 24, 1979

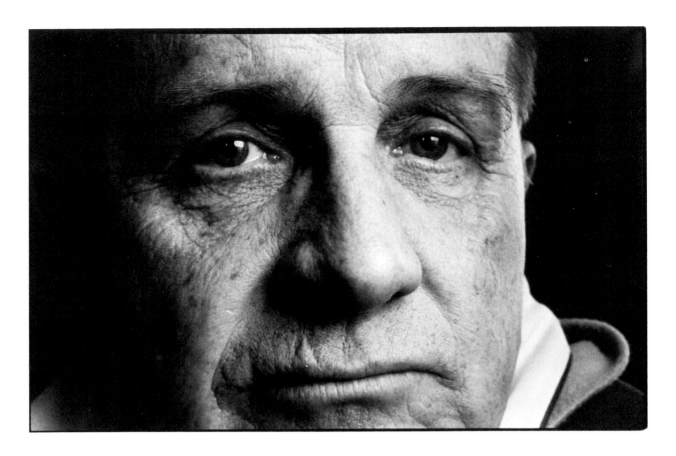

EDWIN MacPHEE:

*The angina starts with pain in my left arm and slowly spreads up the arm, across the chest and—in severe cases—up through the jaws over to the right shoulder. It squeezes and squeezes and I get short of breath.*

BARBARA MacPHEE:

*I can even see you turn grey. But still, if someone were to ask you how you felt then, you'd take a nitroglycerin and say, "Oh, fine."*

January 24, 1979

EDWIN MacPHEE:

*Well, you know, I just have to pop a little nitroglycerin under the tongue, wait a minute, and the pain's gone; everything's okay. I always take a nitro as soon as I get the pain or before doing something that might bring on the pain. I take one on arising in the morning at 5:30, just contemplating the movement of washing my face. About a quarter of six, I take 40 milligrams of Inderol and I put two inches of nitroglycerin paste on my leg; all those pills and paste applications are repeated every six hours. At eight o'clock in the morning, I take one tablespoon of potassium, one half a tablet of Lasix, and three digoxin. I also take between ten and fifteen nitroglycerin tablets a day. My alarm clock wakes me up at night to take my pills at three a.m.*

January 24, 1979

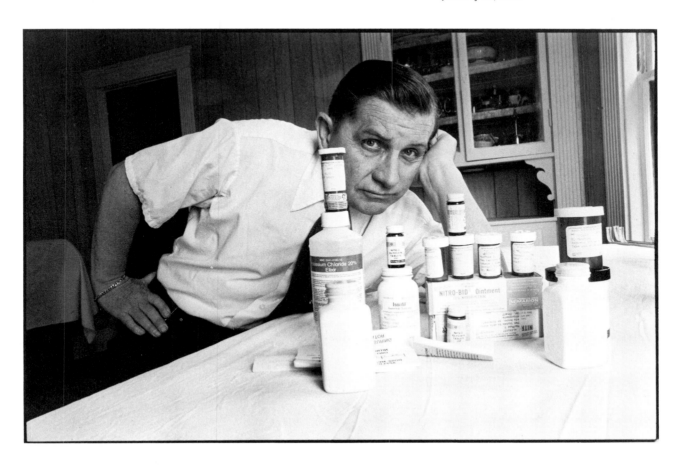

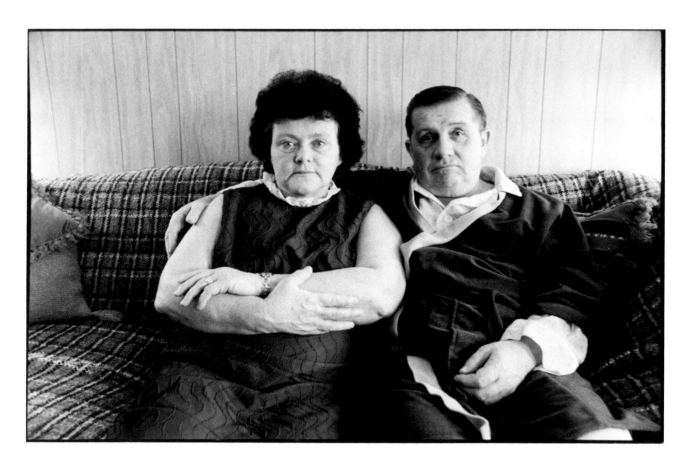

EDWIN MacPHEE:

*I just can't keep up anymore. Even in speaking I can't overdo it because that could bring on angina. If I quicken my pace to keep up with a friend, that will bring on angina—so I usually go for walks by myself. We very seldom attend social functions and even our sex life is at a standstill: a sexual arousal will bring on angina. So you sort of turn off the spigot.*

January 24, 1979

BARBARA MacPHEE:

*About two months ago I told one of the doctors that my husband and I were planning on taking a trip in the summer. He said, "Well you can keep on planning, but I don't think he is going to be around to go on any trip this summer." I told my husband what the doctor had said and he sort of passed it off at the time saying, "I know how bad my heart is, he doesn't have to tell me." But I think it convinced him to have the operation.*

February 6, 1979

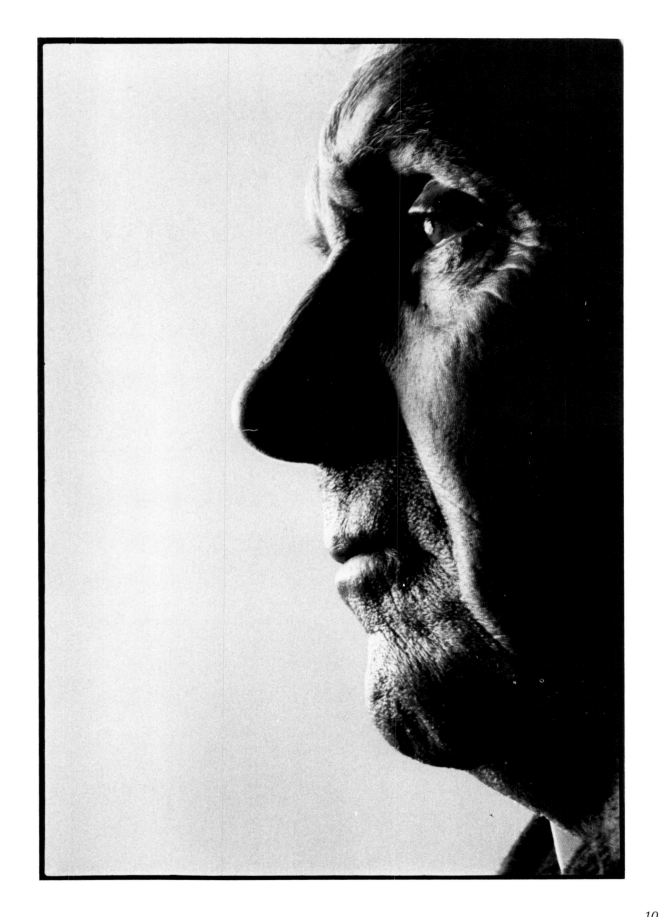

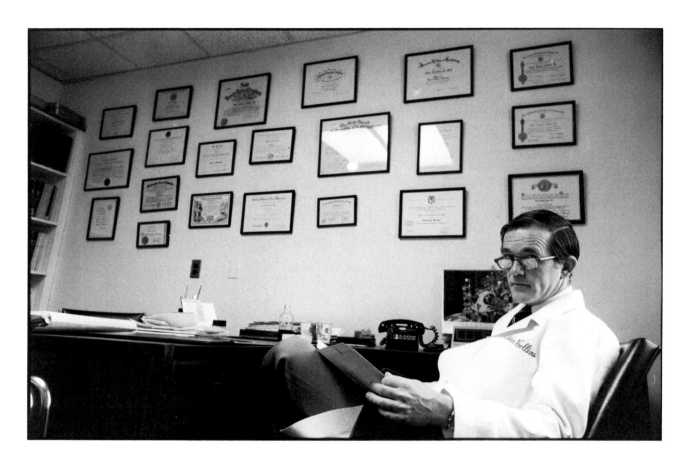

DR. COLLINS:

*Mr. MacPhee's disease is so severe that he has essentially total blockage of his main coronary arteries—we would consider that to be a very hazardous way to exist. Now it's possible that an operation to change his coronary blood flow might make his life more comfortable and longer, but there's a risk in trying to do this: he might lose his life.*

*His risk, in fact, is six or seven times the risk of the average person undergoing this operation. With such a large risk the average person might shy away from such a procedure; but when a person feels terrible, he's not so shy.*

January 31, 1979

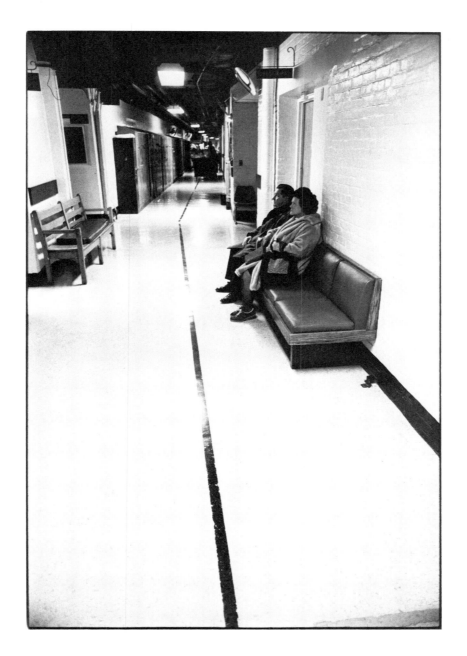

EDWIN MacPHEE:

*I know Dr. Collins and his fine team will do an excellent job and practically eliminate the angina for me. I feel very confident that everything is going to turn out well. Could I be overdoing my confidence in this surgical team? I keep saying that I'm confident in Dr. Collins because you have to be confident. So I'm going to do it and it's going to be great.*

January 24, 1979

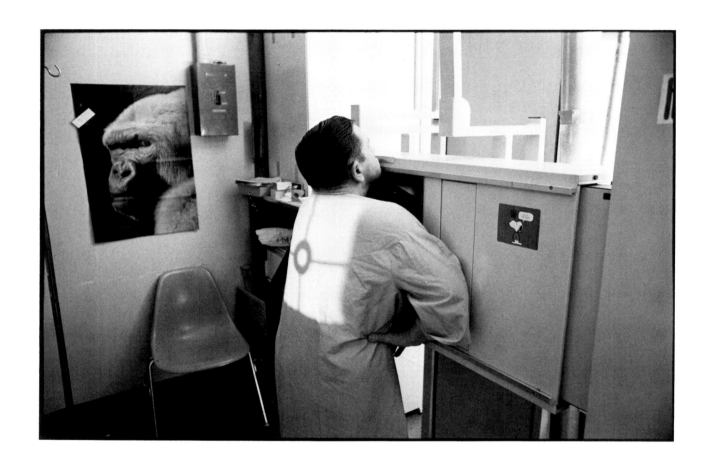

EDWIN MacPHEE:
*The most difficult time was lying up there on the ward waiting to go.*
*We were saying "so long" to each other.*

February 6, 1979

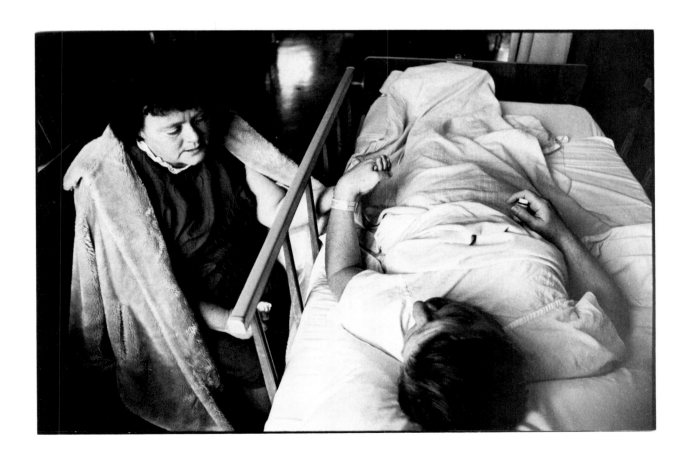

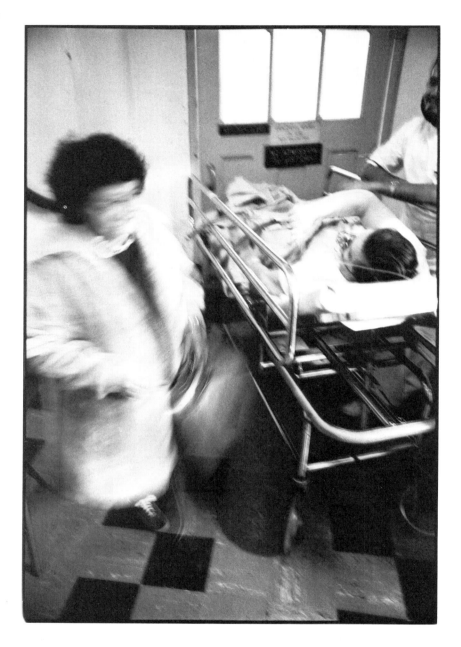

BARBARA MacPHEE:

*I knew how bad his heart was and I didn't think he was ever going to come out of it. I was trying to think how I would ever go on without him, and he kept saying to me there's still time to pull back, we don't have to have this operation.*

February 6, 1979

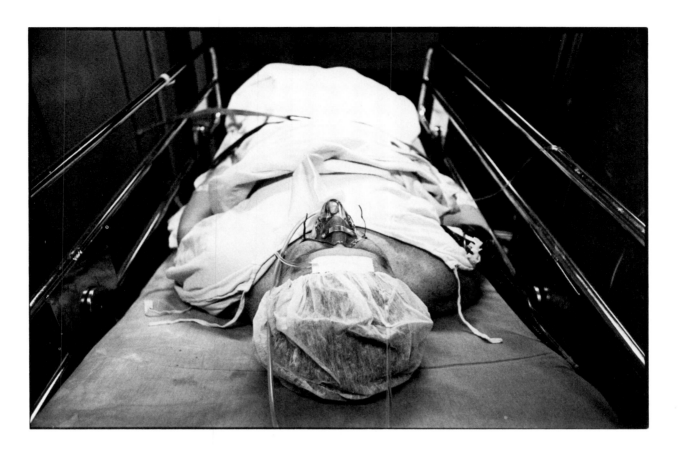

LIBBY BATTIT:
(cardio-thoracic nurse-clinician)

*I think most people fear any kind of surgery. A certain amount of
fear is normal and isn't going to disappear until they have the surgery
behind them.*

January 31, 1979

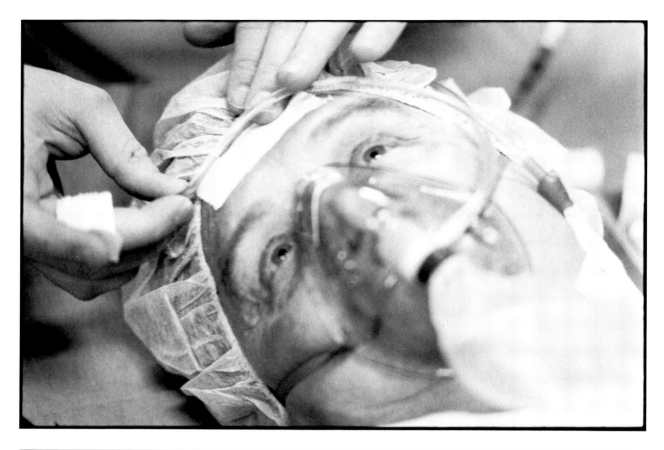

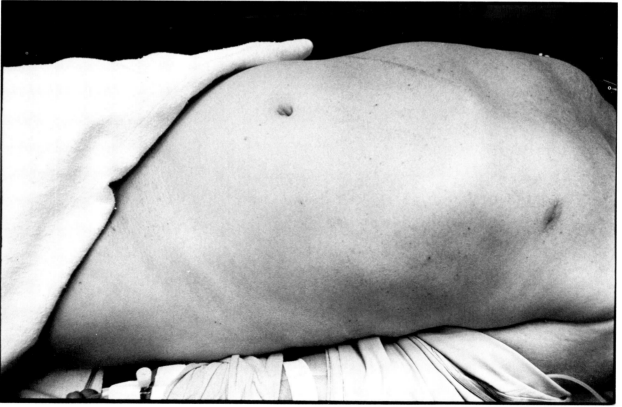

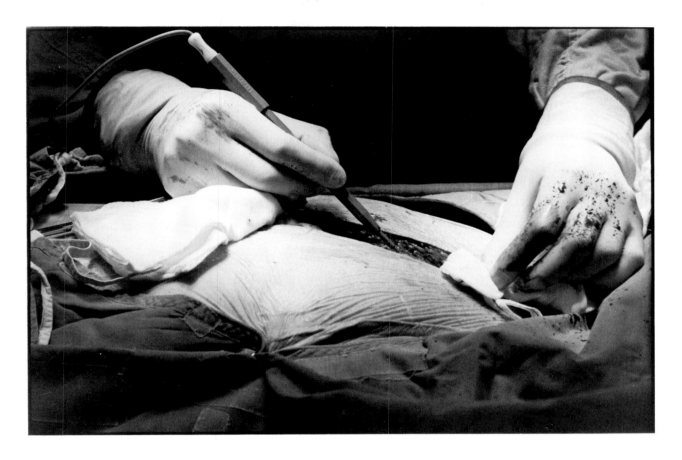

EDWIN MacPHEE:
*There's a risk and that's what you think about, that's what shakes
you up. Am I going to get up off the table? Will my heart—what's left
of my heart—withstand the situation? That's the question in my mind.*

January 24, 1979

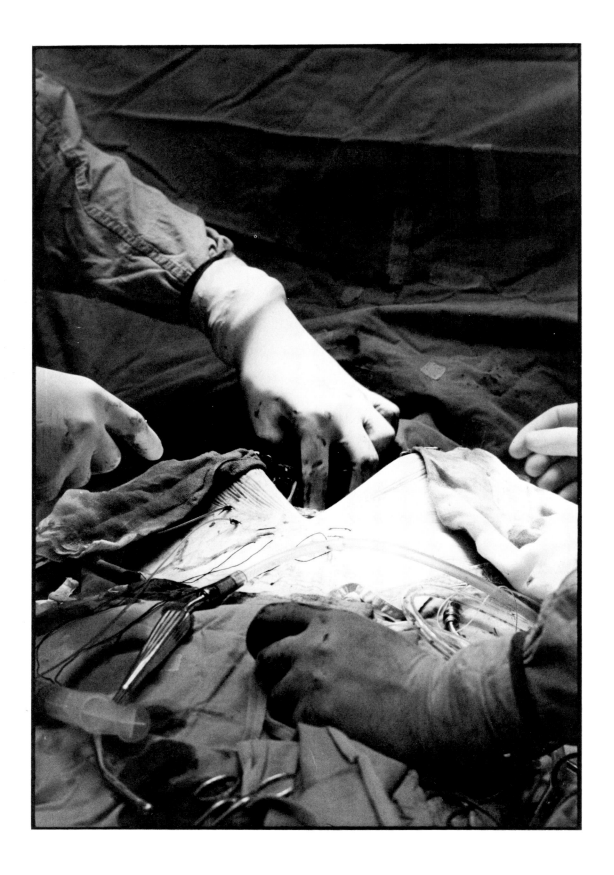

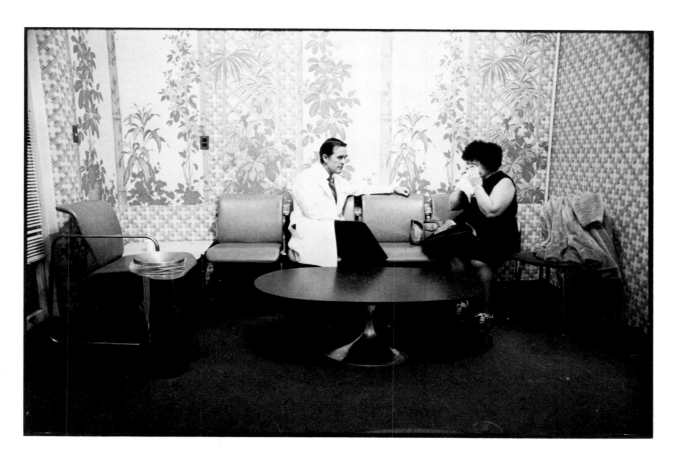

DR. COLLINS:

*When speaking to relatives after the operation, we try to be as calm and cool as possible, without being either unduly optimistic or alarmingly pessismistic. Since relatives don't have the background necessary to understand a disease process in exactly the same fashion the physician understands it, the physician has to be a little careful in his technique of telling the truth. I found it very easy to talk to Mrs. MacPhee because she had lost one husband in the past so she knew that such things happen and could happen again. I told her that we had not made her husband perfect, but we had made him considerably better.*

*The good physician knows that his work—which may appear terribly complicated to the layperson or patient—is really made up of simple parts. It's the same type of knowledge that separates the audience from the magician.*

February 8, 1979

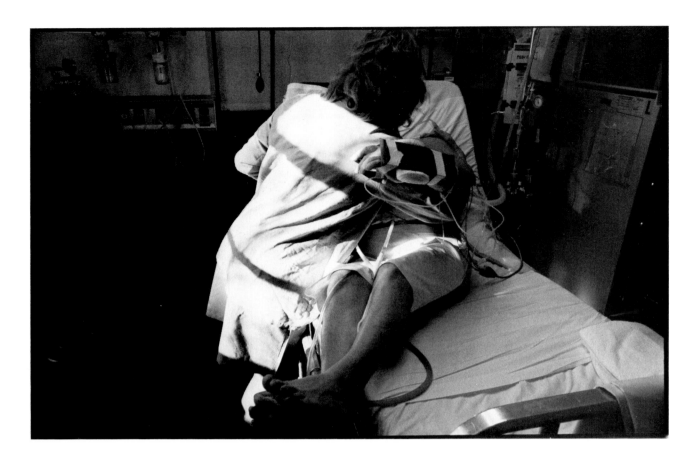

LIBBY BATTIT:
*For the first 24 hours after surgery he still had a lot of the morphine in his system. But by the second post-operative day the morphine had worn off and he became aware of really feeling weak and tired. He hit what we had warned him of: the post-operative slump. Everything was a big effort for him and we were constantly bombarding him with people: nurses, cardiologists, Dr. Collins, the residents, x-ray technicians, nurses who drew blood and put in IV's, EKG technicians, and even the cleaning staff.*

February 7, 1979

EDWIN MacPHEE:
*I may have said this before, but the staff at this hospital, from the outset to the present moment, has been tremendous, and I find that by just listening and doing what the staff explains and tells you, you have no problems at all.*

February 8, 1979

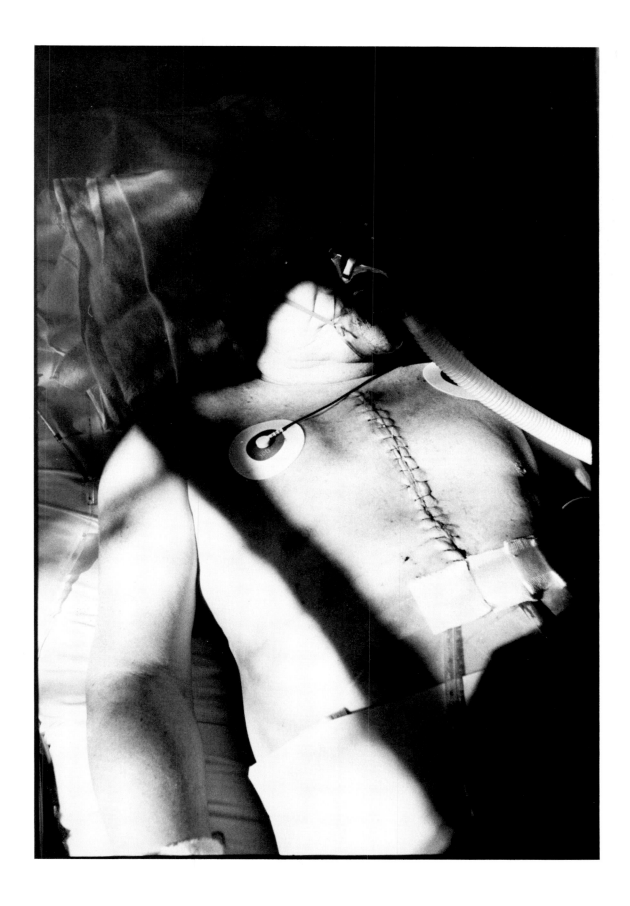

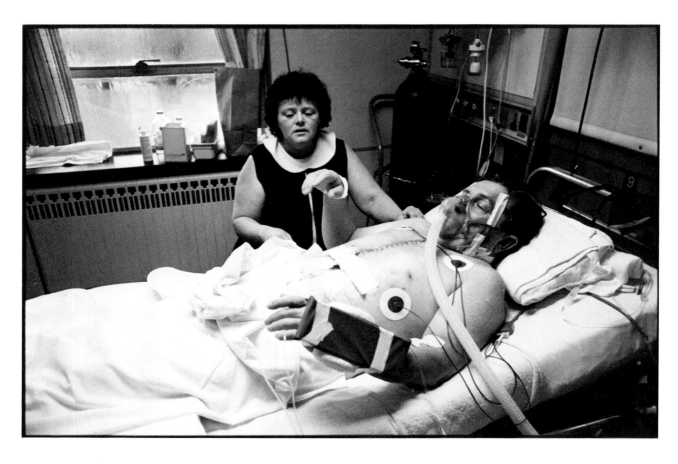

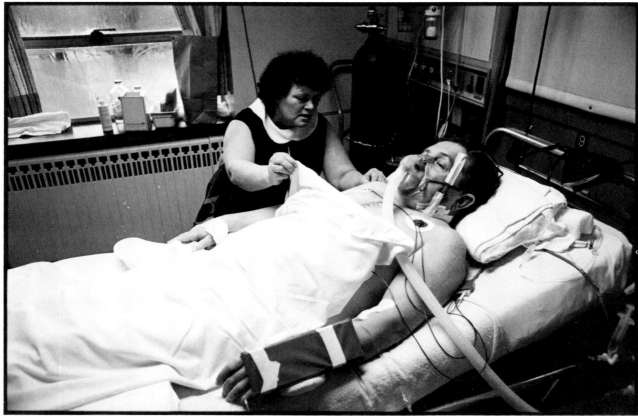

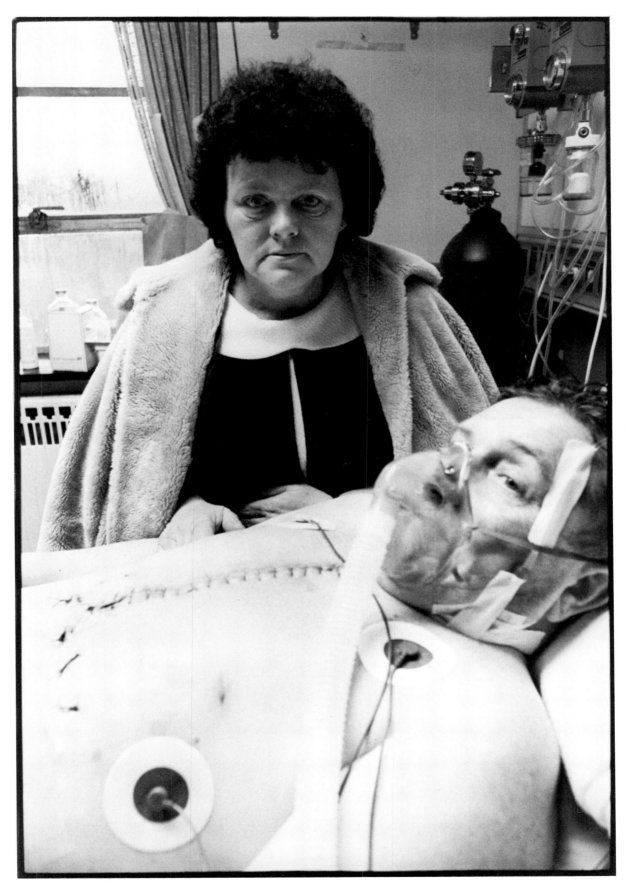

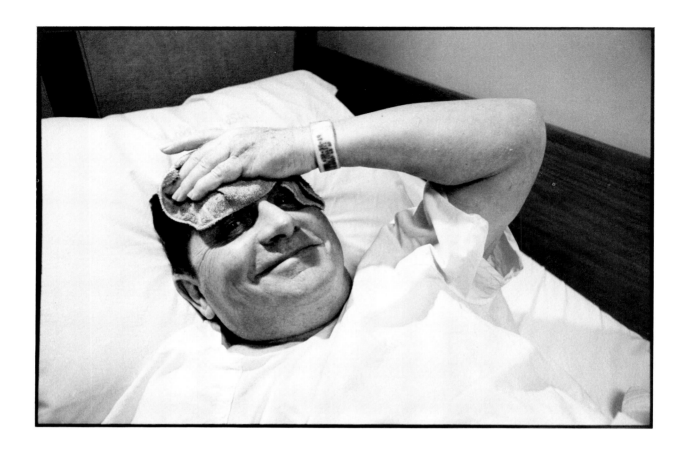

BARBARA MacPHEE:

*Of course, I've been tired, but I've had a feeling inside me of happiness and joy at having this done and taken care of. I could holler hooray! Those severe attacks of angina looked like a dead-end street, but now I can see the tunnel wide open at the end and hopefully I'm going to walk right out through it.*

February 9, 1979

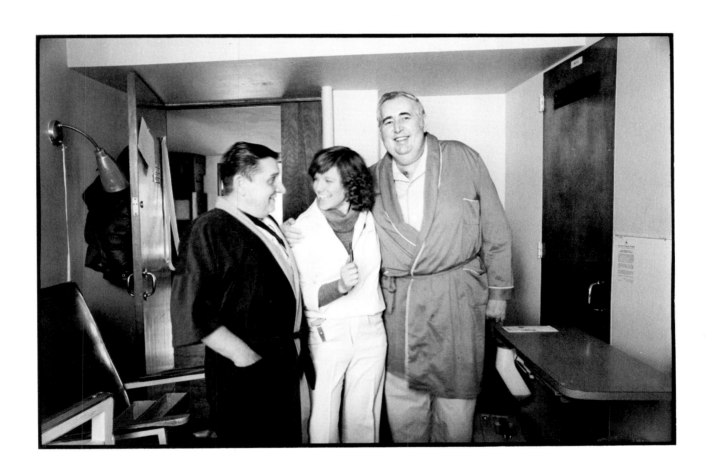

EDWIN MacPHEE:
*I feel so good to have this rebirth, another chance. I know I'm happy,
I know I have no pain. I don't know how long my life will be,
however long it is I know I'm going to enjoy every second of it.*

RICHARD CAMP:
(a fellow patient)
*People seem to be a lot friendlier with each other here because they don't want to be afraid, afraid of leaving their families, afraid of death.*

February 12, 1979

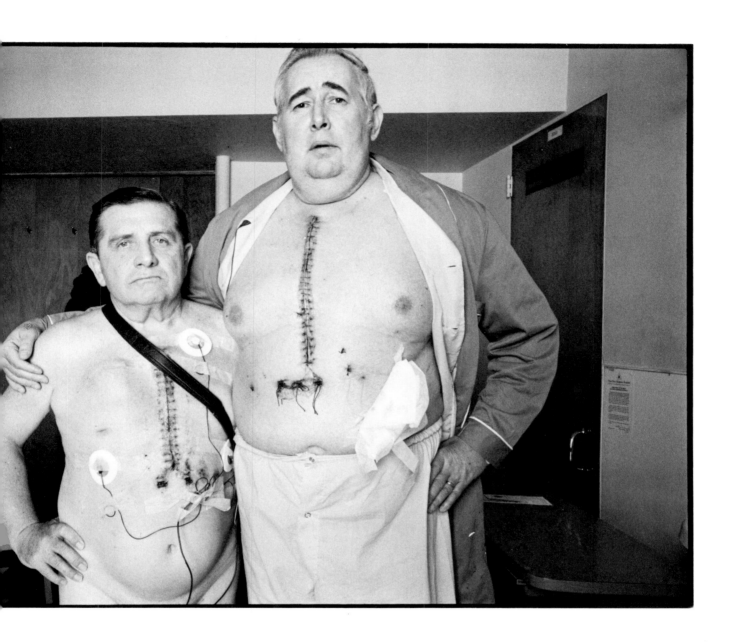

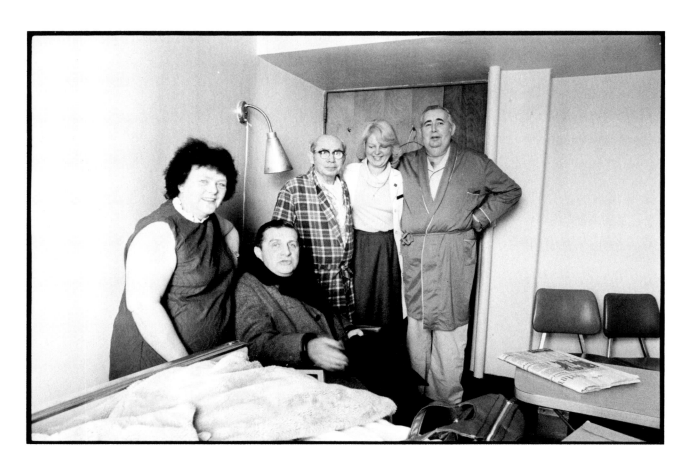

BARBARA MacPHEE:
*I think it does have something to do with the surgery: he was so keyed up before it, and he really thought he was going to die during the operation. When he came out of it, he was so relieved that the operation was over, no pain, everything was so great, and he was just so happy.*

February 28, 1979

BARBARA MacPHEE:
*When he came out of the hospital after his surgery his eyes were all glittering and really big—exactly the way they were when he used to have a drink. He was very excited, talking very fast and louder than usual. He used to have a drinking problem but he didn't give this part of his history to the doctors because he didn't want them to know he did all these crazy things. He told me not to dare mention it.*

February 21, 1979

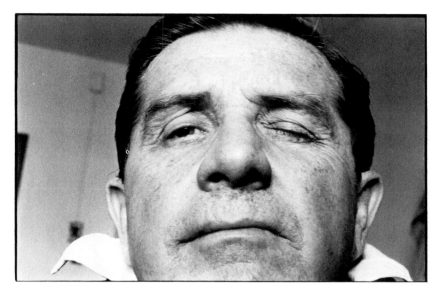

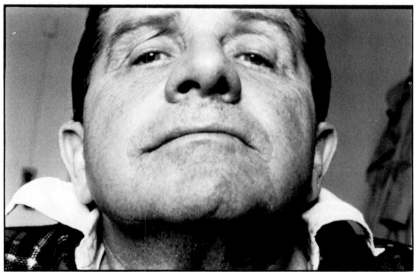

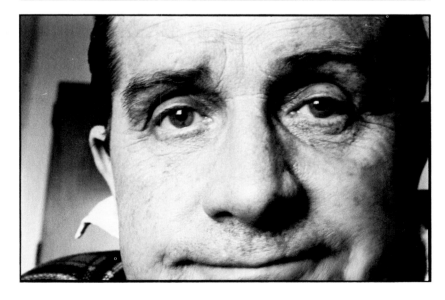

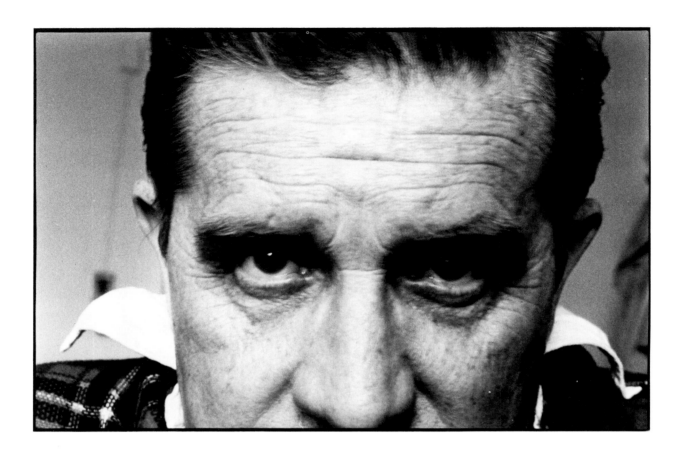

DR. JOAN FLURI:
(Mr. MacPhee's Cardiologist at Veterans Hospital)

*The day of his discharge from Peter Bent Brigham he was quite jovial and euphoric at having come through surgery with the odds so high against him. On the third day after discharge he was making inappropriate telephone calls to patients at three o'clock in the morning. It may be normal to be very happy, but not to the point of losing good judgment—and certainly it would not be good judgment to call a patient who is sick at three o'clock in the morning. His excessive euphoria became a problem that needed psychiatric consultation and arrangements were made to admit him to the Veterans Hospital.*

Febraury 21, 1979

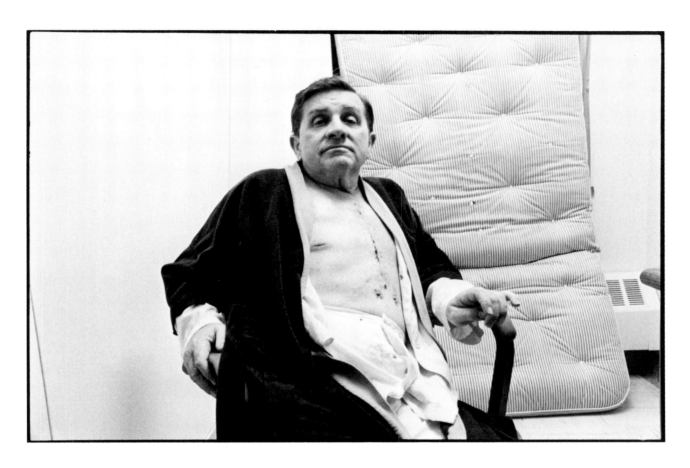

EDWIN MacPHEE:

*I can't put it out of my mind. When I was in the service, I was 18, in the United States infantry overseas with Patton's Third Army. One night, prior to attack, we went out and looked over the attack area. Coming back through some brush, my glasses flipped off and I couldn't see well, so I told the Captain, "I can't lead the squad because I don't have my glasses." "You're a coward," he said. I said, "No, I'm not a coward." So I went and led it. Two of my men got killed, two of my dearest friends, two good soldiers. If I had died during the surgery I would have seen them in heaven. They would have said, "You told us to go there and we got killed." I know how it wasn't my fault, and those boys are in a better place, and they love me. One got it right between the eyes and the other right through the heart—right through the front of his chest, just where I had my thorax cut by the great Dr. Collins.*

February 21, 1979

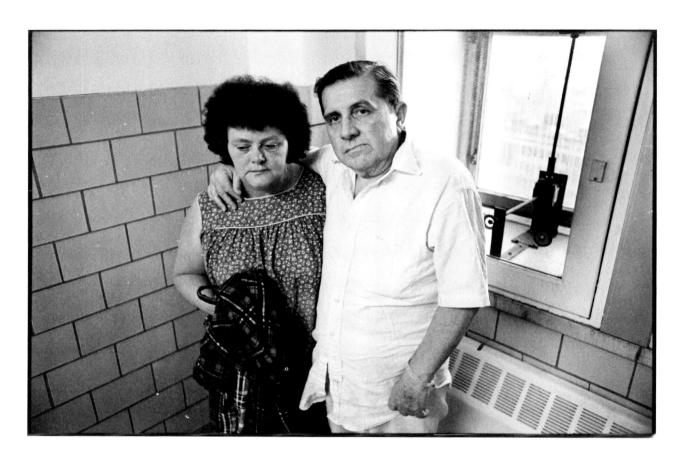

BARBARA MacPHEE:

*This is the worst he's ever been: his eyes look strange and his speech is very slurred. I really don't know what is happening. I wonder if he's going to come out of it or if he's going to be like this forever. I am sorry he ever had the operation. If I had had any idea this was going to happen, I would have talked him out of it.*

February 28, 1979

DR. JOAN FLURI:
*Five days later I was surprised to see him. His affect had changed considerably: he was now very depressed. I think the depression is more appropriate than the euphoria. Any of us in approaching a major stress situation like surgery get geared up for it; and then we're so relieved that it's over, and that we have met the challenge, that we almost fall apart. I think depression is normal following this type of stressful situation. Family members also go through the stress of worrying, hoping, and praying—and they can expect to have some letdown afterwards, too.*

February 28, 1979

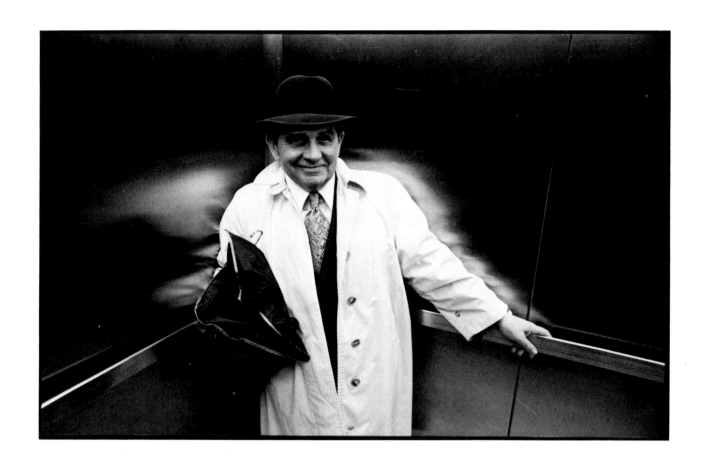

DR. STUART GOLDMAN:
(Psychiatrist)

*Prior to the operation Mr. MacPhee was able to deny a lot of sad feelings from his loss of ability to do many things. What he had been able to say was, that it feels great to be alive and he feels wonderful. Clearly there were things that were not wonderful about his life.*

*I think the extreme stress of realizing that he might die on the operating table during cardiac surgery was too much to deny and that stress triggered this episode. Chances are now he'll leave the hospital, and barring some unforeseen stresses, not have more difficulties.*

March 7, 1979

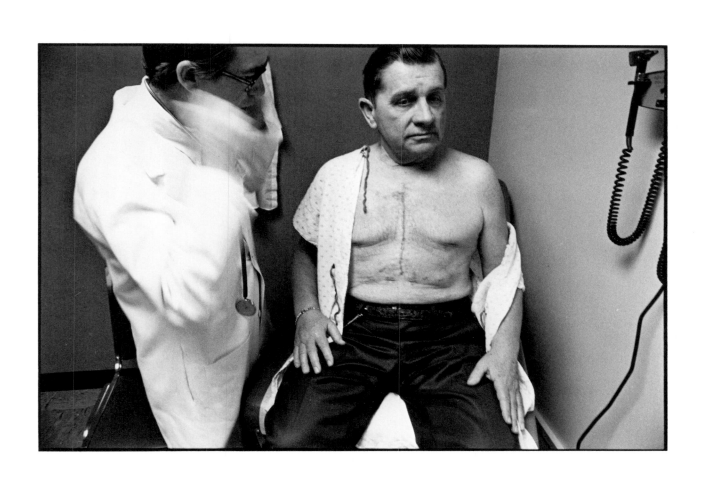

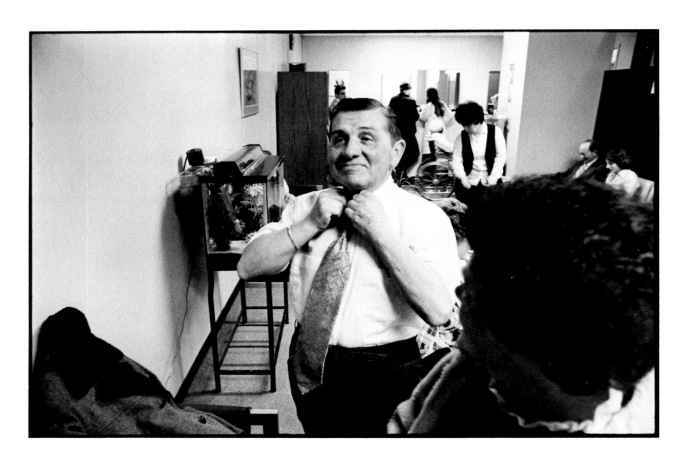

EDWIN MacPHEE:
*I just had my checkup with Dr. Collins and he said everything looks fine, and I'm coming along nicely. I told him I had no problems. I explained how I had a little angina but I thought it was due to the cold weather or walking too rapidly. It's just a little tickle in the shoulder.*

March 29, 1979

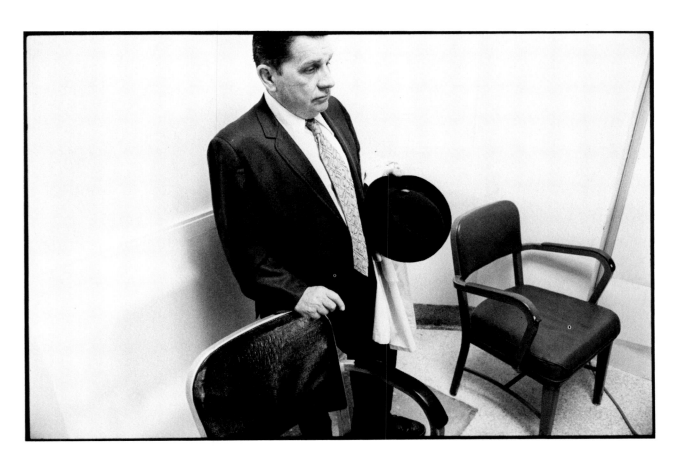

DR. JOAN FLURI:
*He seems too accepting of his pain, just like pre-operatively when he
told me everything was fine—and he had taken 50 nitroglycerin pills
that day! To me the new onset of angina now is very disturbing, and I
think that if someone went through all that he's gone through and
had recurrent chest pain, he should be either angry or very sad about
the whole thing and have a lot of questions about it. He looks a little
saddened but he is still thinking that things are pretty good.*

April 12, 1979

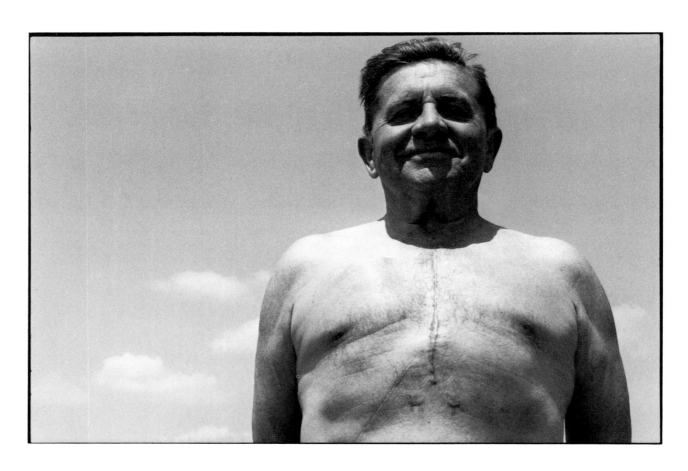

EDWIN MacPHEE:
*I feel so good now. It's absolutely wonderful. I get out and walk two or three miles along the beach. If I take things at a very slow pace everything seems to work out fine. No problems.*

May 6, 1979

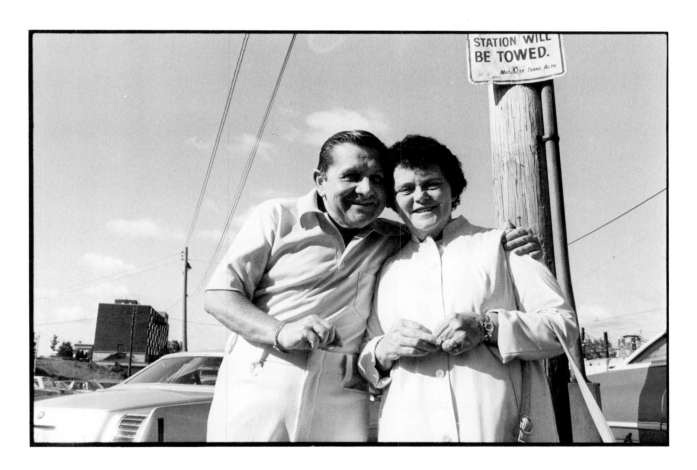

EDWIN MacPHEE:

When I used to get those terrible attacks of angina I felt that one of them was just going to take me out of it. I'm not as nervous now.

Barbara and I seem to discuss things more. We talk about things we see in the newspaper and current events, where before it was just a constant concern about my health.

And today we're off on our little vacation. You know, the one they said I wouldn't live for.

August 15, 1979

137

EDWIN MacPHEE:

*Now I don't have that constant concern about how long I am going to be here or whether it is going to be today, tomorrow, or how long.*

August 15, 1979

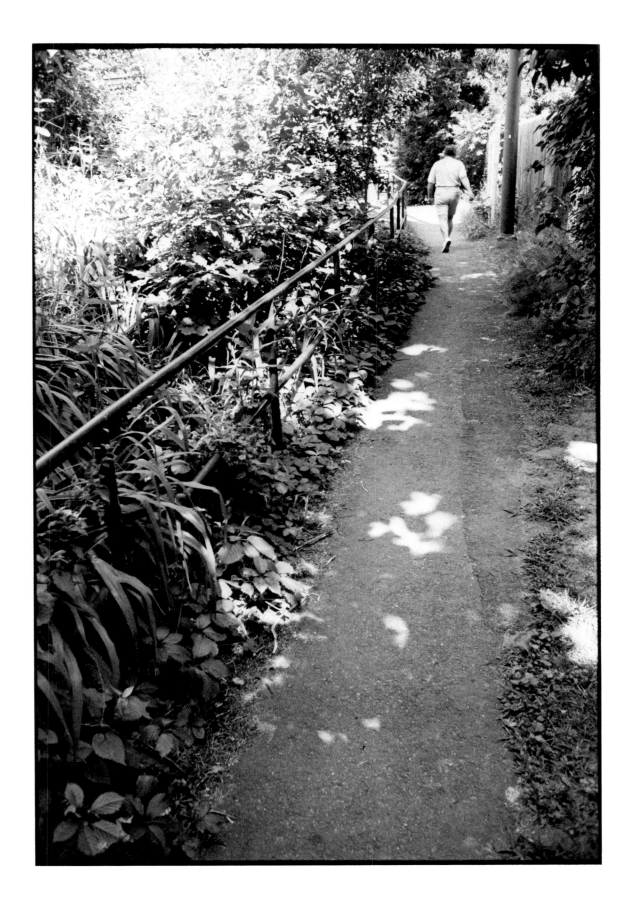

# Jeanne McLaughlin

Jeanne McLaughlin is a licensed practical nurse. She earned this degree in 1966 when illness had forced her husband into early retirement and made it necessary for her to support her family. On October 25, 1976, she underwent a mastectomy for breast cancer. Two weeks after her surgery her husband moved back to their mobile home in Florida where the McLaughlins had previously spent their winters. Jeanne McLaughlin joined her husband in Florida ten weeks later after her surgical scars had healed. Subsequent tests showed no evidence that her tumor had spread beyond her breast, and she has continued to work as a nurse.

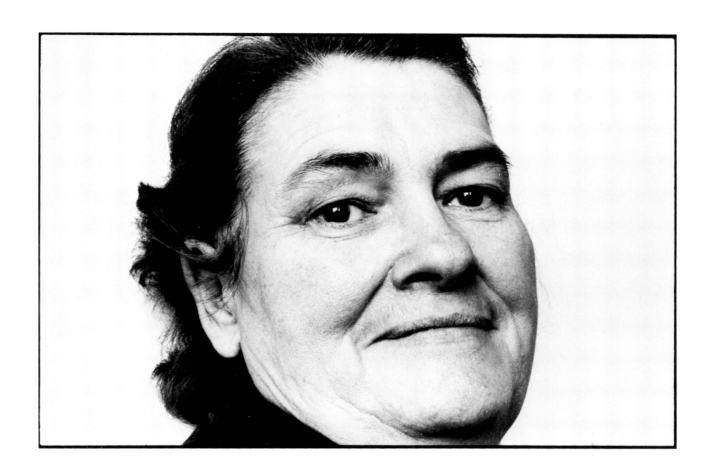

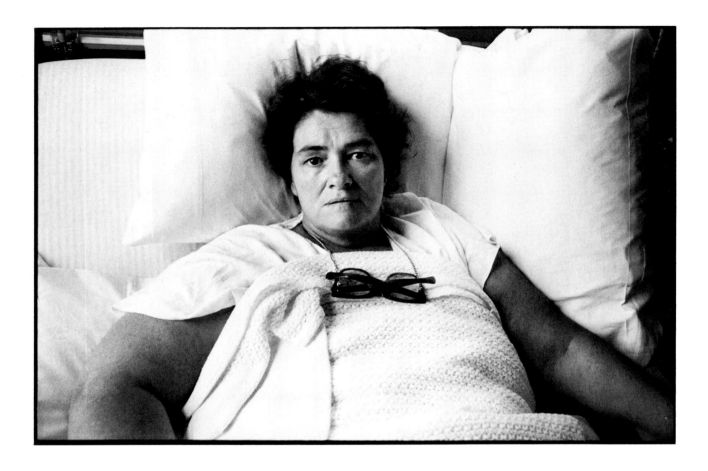

JEANNE McLAUGHLIN:

*I first felt the lump in my breast one day when I was taking a
bath. Then, about two weeks later, I reexamined myself and
noticed that it was growing. At the time my husband was too ill
for me to take care of it, so I let it go for about six weeks before I
went to the doctor.*

*They took me right in, gave me an emergency appointment,
and then had me see the surgeon. He said at that time he
thought it was cancerous, that it would need operating.*

October 26, 1976

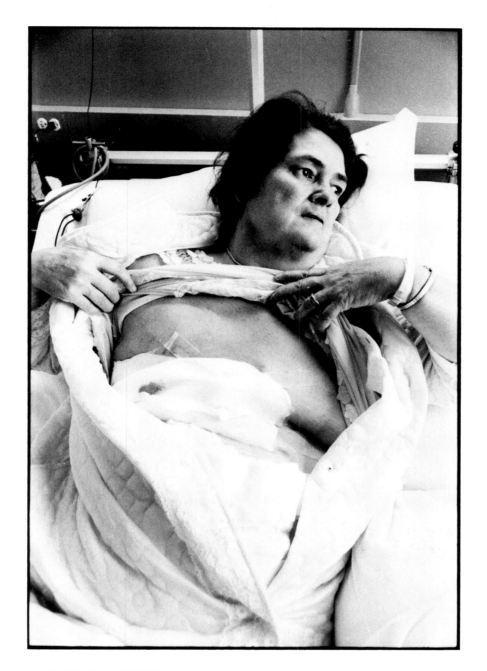

JEANNE McLAUGHLIN:

*It really didn't hit me when the doctor told me in the clinic. I said to myself, he's making a mistake. And that's what I let myself think until I got home. When I got home it really hit me like a ton of bricks. I cried most of that night and most of the next day before I was even able to think about it rationally. And then I was angry, bitterly, bitterly angry...angry at everyone and everything.*

*For days, I was depressed, despondent. My first thought was suicide: why go through all that pain and suffering if you're going to die anyway?*

October 28, 1976

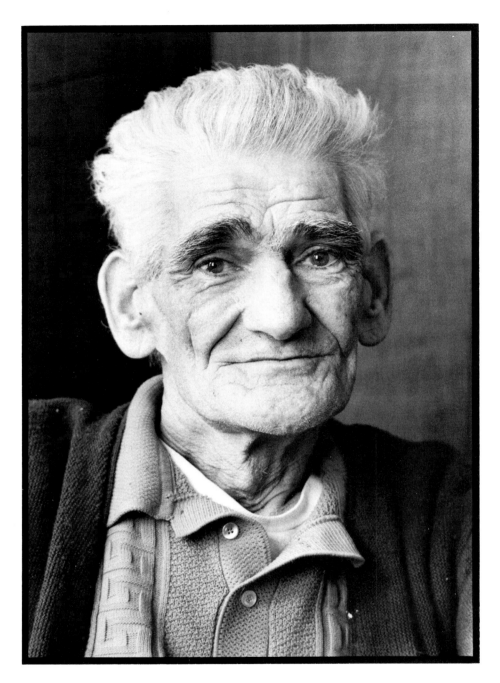

JEANNE McLAUGHLIN:

*I'd step in front of a train. I really did consider it very seriously. The only reason I didn't do it is that I have a sick husband to care for. Why should I punish him for something that he has no control over? And it would be punishing him if I left him in the care of others. We married for better or for worse. It's my duty to take care of him—he took care of me all these years. We've been married 38 years last Monday, and he gave me the best years of his life. This was one of the reasons that I decided that I would go on with my life and do the best I could.*

October 30, 1976

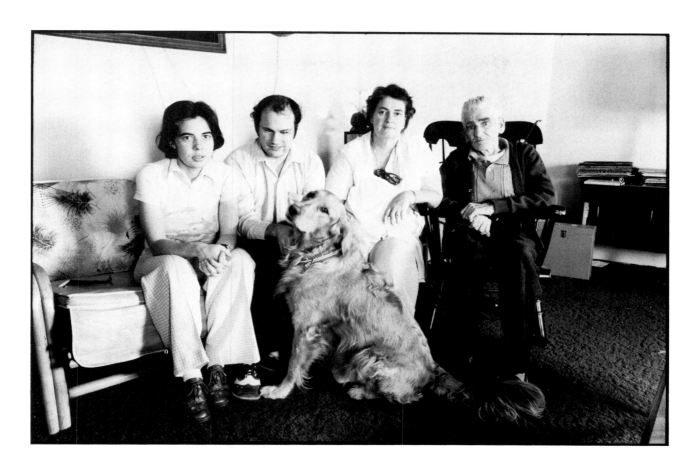

JEANNE McLAUGHLIN:
*There were a lot of things to think about.*

*My husband has been sick off and on for the last six to eight years with emphysema, and very sick this past summer.*

*My daughter here in South Boston is not badly retarded, but retarded enough so that she can't handle illness and can't handle excessive cooking. She gets by. She does very well. She's 29 this year and she's equivalent to about a 17- to 19-year old and just as flighty.*

*Her husband is blind. He is in his last year of college and planning to go on to be a social worker for the blind. He is a lovely man, and they get along fine together.*

October 30, 1976

JEANNE McLAUGHLIN:

*When I began to accept that I would have to have something done, I put a lot of thought into deciding what type of operation I would have. With a simple mastectomy they do not remove the muscles. And if you have the muscles, you're not as debilitated and you can use your arm sooner. With a radical mastectomy they remove arm and chest muscles so I would be laid up at least three months. With a simple mastectomy, I would return to work after three weeks.*

*And I have to get back to work quickly. My husband will not allow me to apply for welfare and there is no other way to support myself. The doctor preferred the radical because he felt he could do better for me with that. He said the decision was strictly up to me. But when I told him I wanted the simple, I had a feeling he was angry with me. He didn't really say anything—he just turned and walked away.*

*If I had been in circumstances where I could have made the other decision, and been able to stay at home until I could get well...I would have felt that I had done better for myself, that I would have given myself a better chance of life. This way I'm not sure I have.*

October 28, 1976

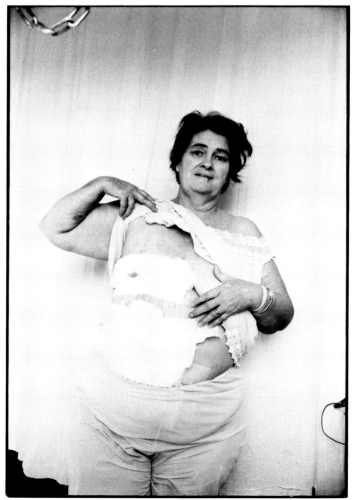

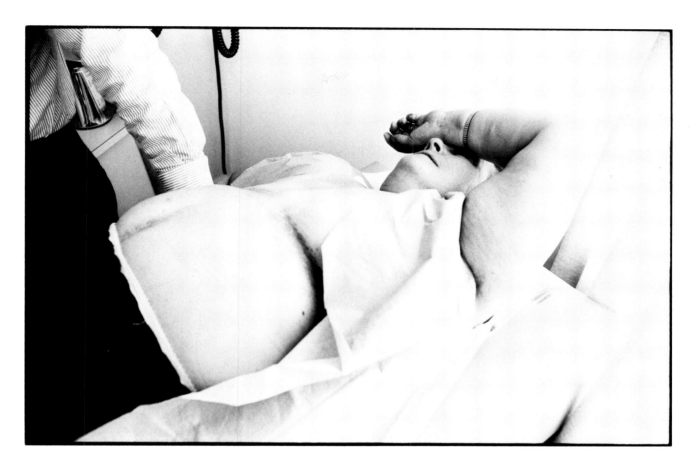

JEANNE McLAUGHLIN:

*That first day, right after the operation, I had feelings of desolation, a feeling of abandonment, a feeling that I no longer wanted to live. I had made up my mind that if nobody cared enough to come for me that day, that if I had to take the streetcar home, I was going to go into the subway and do away with myself.*

*Real fear stopped me from doing it when I realized I might still be alive afterward. Then the pains and anguish and the frustration that I would have to go through would be even worse. I might be bedridden or paralyzed and still be alive.*

*I don't even think about it any more. I realize that it was foolish and that I really have a lot to give to life. I have a lot that I **want** to give.*

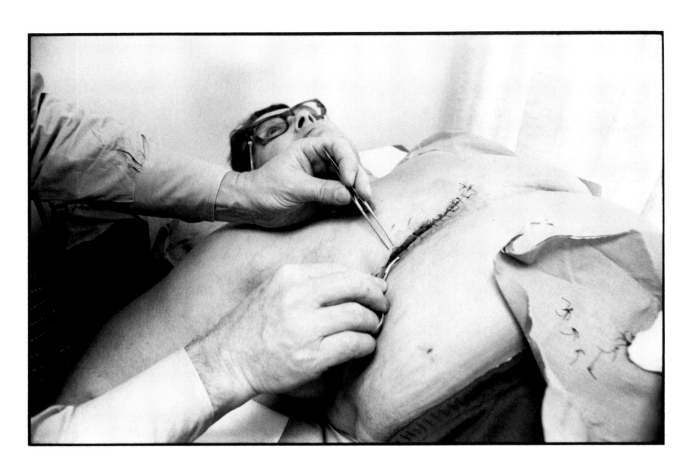

JEANNE McLAUGHLIN:

*I still have resentment and anger to a certain degree...just at life, at the world. Why does all the hardship seem to hit in certain places and certain people? Because someone thinks they are stronger and they can take it?*

November 2, 1976

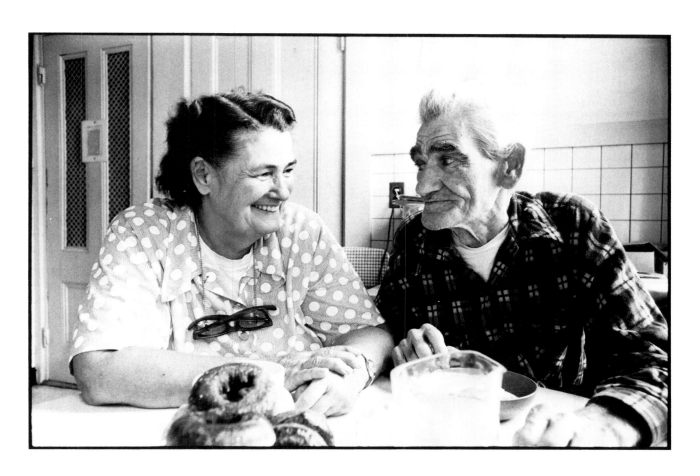

JEANNE McLAUGHLIN:

*But then, you can look around you.*

*And you can always find somebody worse off than you are. So you wonder where does that thinking get you. It's not really very rational.*

*But, then, I wasn't very rational during the last three or four weeks.*

November 4, 1976

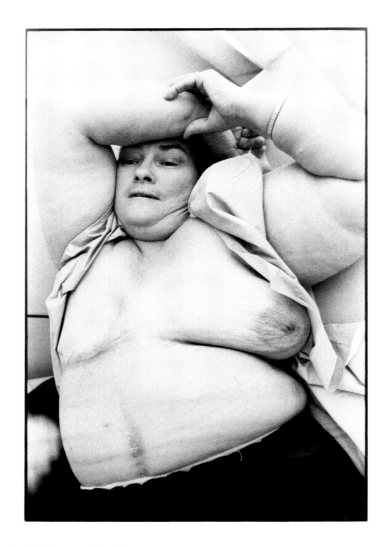

JEANNE McLAUGHLIN:

*My husband had been very, very depressed, angry, and upset.
Of course, when he heard about me he became even more
depressed. Now he's afraid that I'm going to die before him and
leave him with the children. He doesn't want to be with them
unless I'm there.*

*The last doctor that he had insisted on telling him that he had
cancer. I didn't want them to tell him but they did. He's not the
type that can handle it, and this is one of the reasons that he's
so despondent. He's threatened several times to go out the win-
dow. Of course my daughter gets frantic and runs out of the
house. You can't blame her. She has enough problems to handle
as it is.*

*The doctor insisted on telling him, the lung doctor.*

November 4, 1977

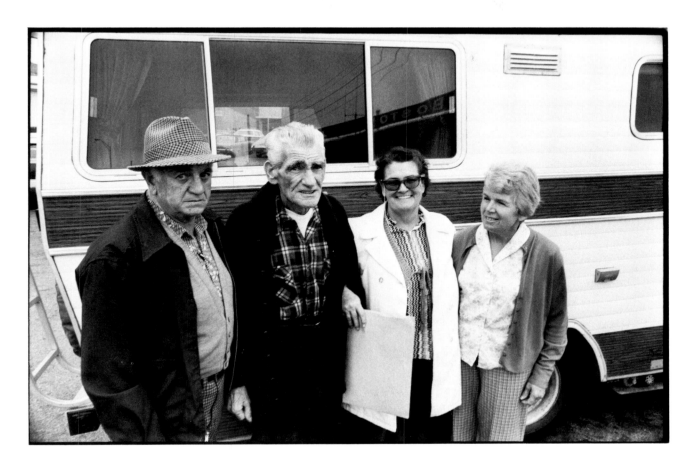

JEANNE McLAUGHLIN:

*He won't talk about it. He won't say anything, so I can't tell you how he's reacting. I don't think he's spoken four dozen words to me except for telling me to leave him alone and let him die. All he talks about is wanting to go back to Florida where it's warm. He is afraid of staying up here in the cold.*

November 4, 1976

JOE:
(A friend of the McLaughlin's)

*Mr. McLaughlin always felt better in Florida, and was very unhappy to come North. When we heard of his...dilemma...his illness...we felt there was only one thing to do. We came up, since he wanted to go to Florida, to take him down.*

November 5, 1976

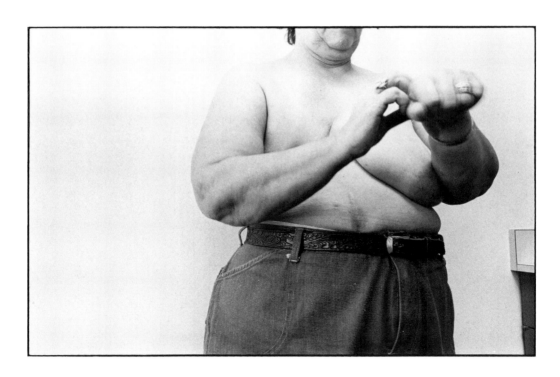

JEANNE McLAUGHLIN:

*But I wonder if some of why he's running to Florida—he claims*
*it's because of the sunshine—is because I've had this operation.*
*He's not a man that ever could take much sickness.*

December 5, 1977

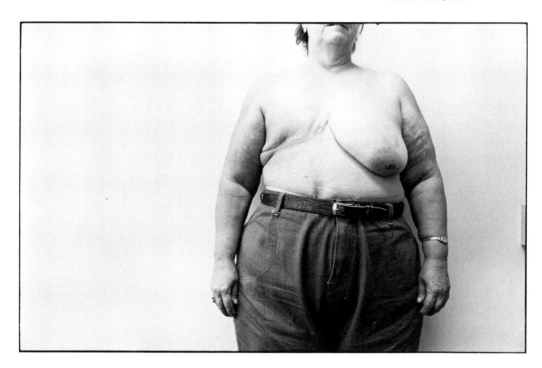

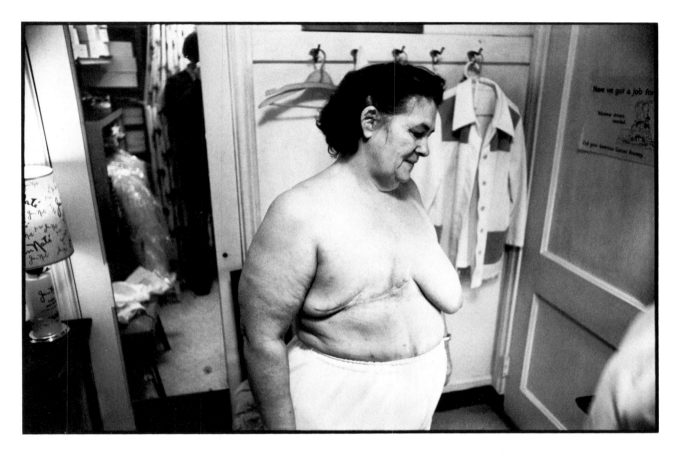

JEANNE McLAUGHLIN:

*When I first went back to work, I felt everyone knew that I had something done, whether they did know it or not. Everyone was looking at me, watching me to see how things fit. I just knew that everyone else knew.*

January 9, 1978

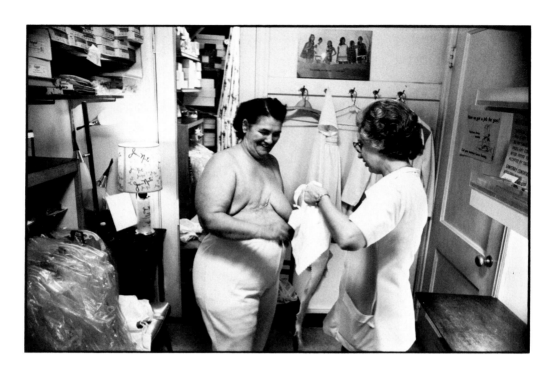

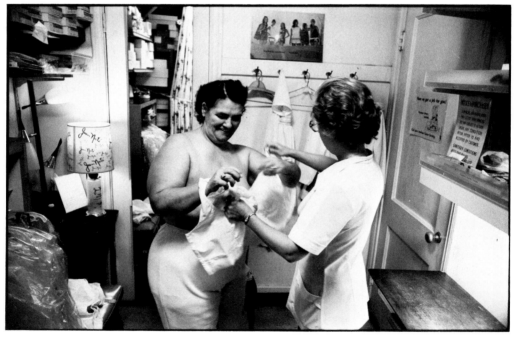

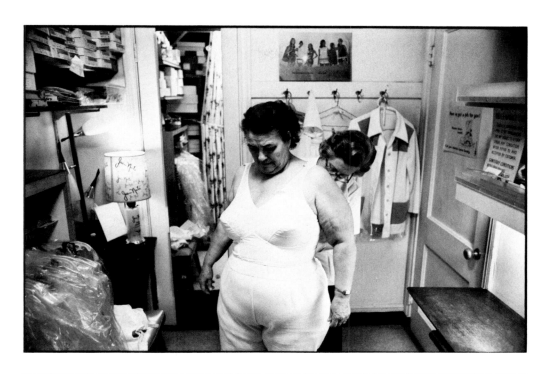

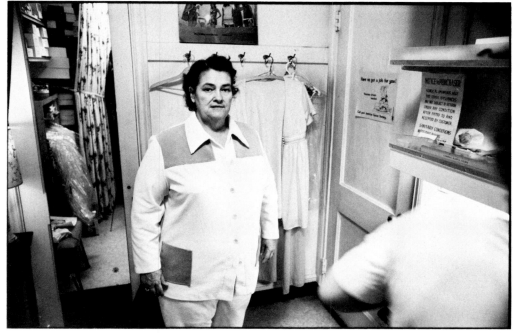

JEANNE McLAUGHLIN:

*Three months*
*For the feeling*
*That I could again be comfortable.*
*And know that I look normal*
*And know that I look all right.*
*And that people*
*Don't know*                                    January 9, 1978

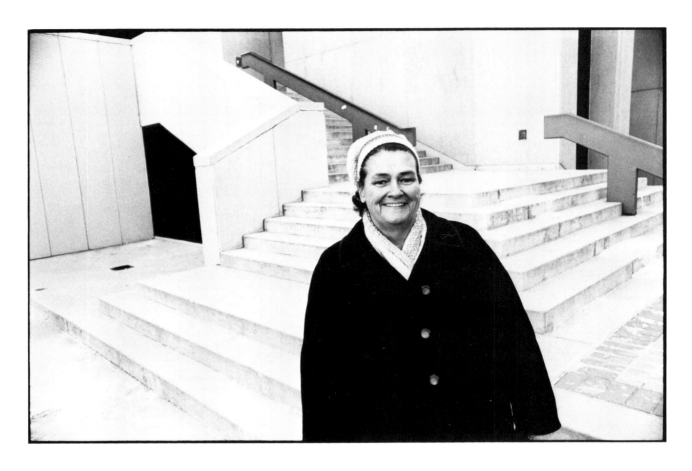

JEANNE McLAUGHLIN:

*If you could only bring it out so that you can talk about it and face it, this is the way to answer it. But we don't want to do that. We want to keep it all to ourselves, and dwell on it, and think about it, and punish ourselves. Why we want to punish ourselves I don't understand...but this is essentially what we are doing.*

December 22, 1976

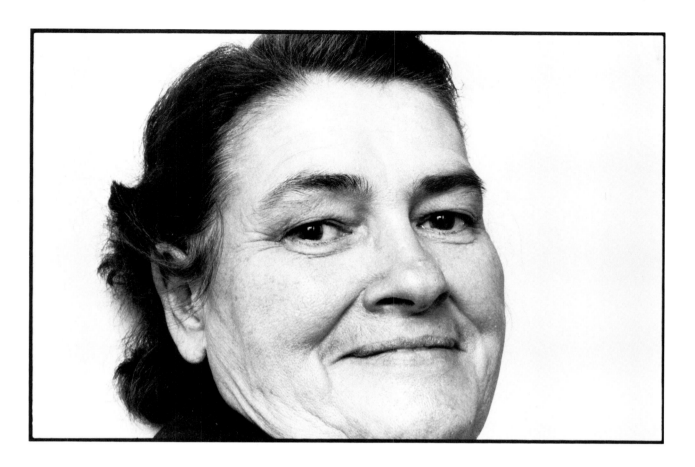

Miami, Florida
January 24, 1977

*Hello Mark,*

*Just a note to let you know all here are well but tired. I do have a job (V.A. Hospital), will start January 31. I found an apartment, three rooms, fair condition, one-and-one-half blocks from that hospital. Jackson Hospital, where Owen will be going, is just across the street from the V.A. Hospital.*

*Owen has improved physically and mentally, attitude is much better. But oh, so much pain.*

*He wanted me to do as I thought right, but was unable to tell me. He had many fears about the doctor's ability to get all of the cancer. He still thinks about it and worries about it being okay.*

*He states he cannot sleep with me yet as he is afraid that in thrashing, he would hurt me physically. He is still unable to look at my surgery. I'm not pushing this part, as I feel less of a woman; I also feel a great loss, an embarrassment that I did not have with you and the doctor. I don't understand this feeling. Sometimes a feeling of not being whole. I know this sounds foolish, but it is real to me.*

*Thanks again and oblige,*
*Jeanne McLaughlin*

# Joel Bruinooge

Joel Bruinooge, 26 years old, worked as a writer and editor in the public relations department of a large insurance company and had been married to Meg Crissara, a pianist, for almost three years when he suffered a stroke on January 13, 1977. The stroke resulted from a blockage in one of the vertebral arteries which supplied blood to parts of his brain, and it caused him to have difficulty with speech and balance. It is very unusual for a stroke to affect men as young as Joel and though his physicians performed a multitude of diagnostic tests, they could find no physiological explanation for why he had the stroke.

He made a gradual recovery and returned to work six weeks after his stroke. On April 22, however, he suffered a heart attack caused by a blockage in one of the arteries that supplied his blood to heart. He was hospitalized for another three weeks and returned to work shortly thereafter. In October 1979 he was still working full-time, having been promoted since his initial illness.

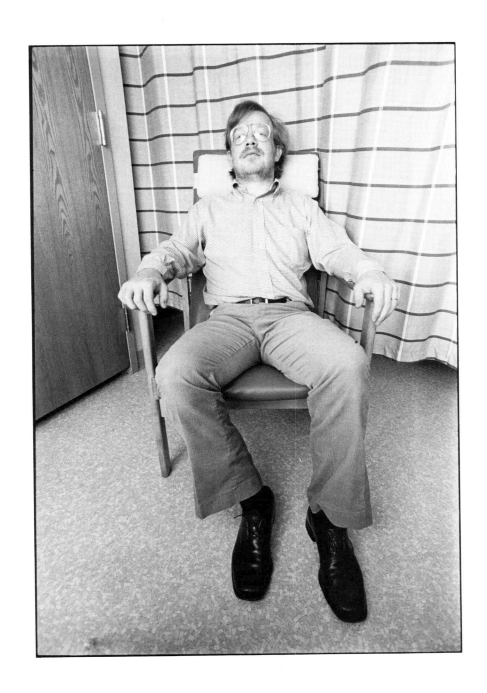

JOEL BRUINOOGE:

*I felt like I had the flu: I was dizzy, mildly nauseated, really tired, and I just wanted to go to bed.*

*At the hospital, it took them a long time to figure out what it was. At first they thought it was a migraine headache. Then they did a brain scan and still didn't know what it was. Then, the next day, they did the angiogram and found the clot.*

*I don't even remember the first two or three days. It's like I was asleep the whole time, and anxious.*

January 25, 1977

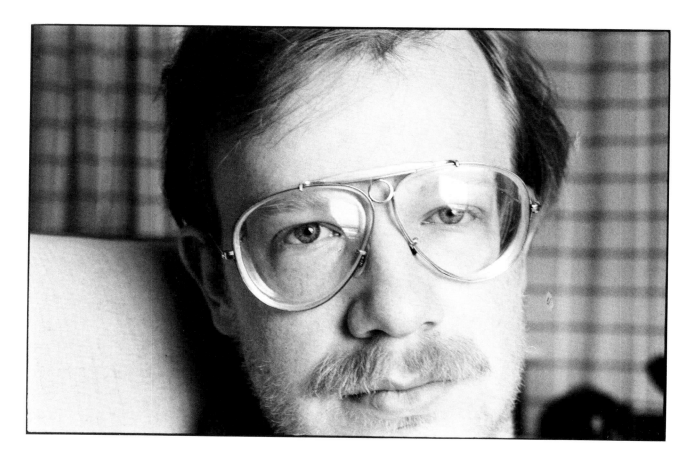

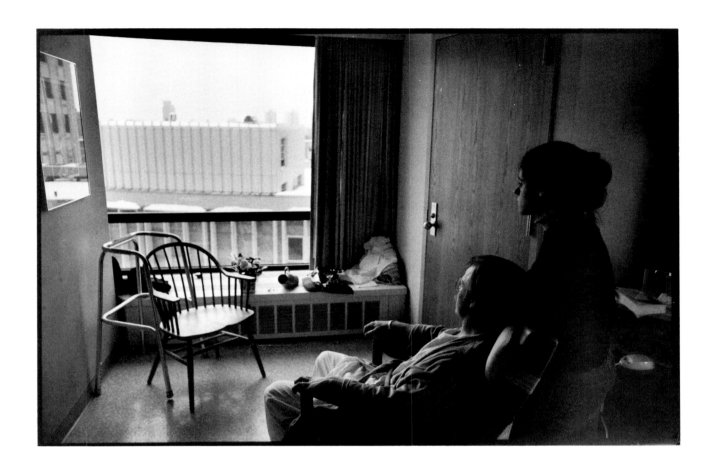

MEG CRISSARA:
(Joel's wife)

In the beginning I was really afraid he was going to die. One of
the doctors said it's either a migraine headache, an aneurysm,
or a brain tumor. He said that so matter of factly, but it sounded
like things were not going to be good at all. I was frightened and
I couldn't sleep.

After they did the angiogram, Dr. Caplan took me into the
solarium and sat me down. He told me it was a vascular occlusion—and I had to ask him what that meant. So he told me Joel
had had a stroke. I couldn't handle it at all. I was petrified and I
just cried a lot. He was really kind, and he stayed with me for a
long time, maybe fifteen minutes, until I was a little better.

January 25, 1977

JON BRUINOOGE:
(Joel's older brother)
*Joel was under a lot of emotional stress. Last Christmas when he got very excited and angry about some inconsequential political topic, he turned completely red and his voice escalated. I said "Jesus Christ, you've gotta calm down, you're gonna have yourself a stroke!"*

*After it happened my immediate concern was, "Is the kid gonna be a vegetable?"*

January 26, 1977

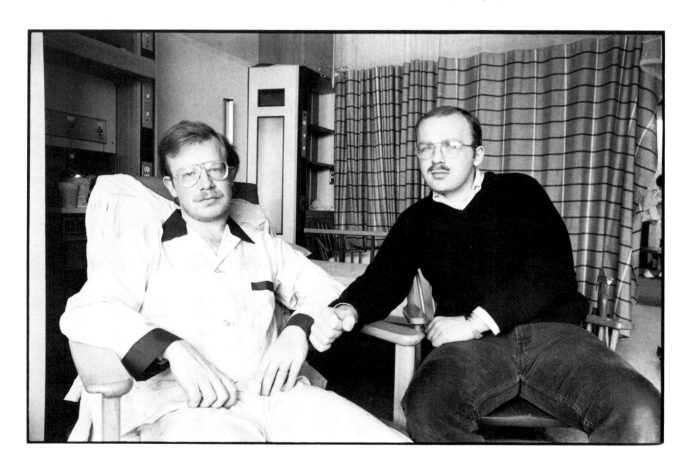

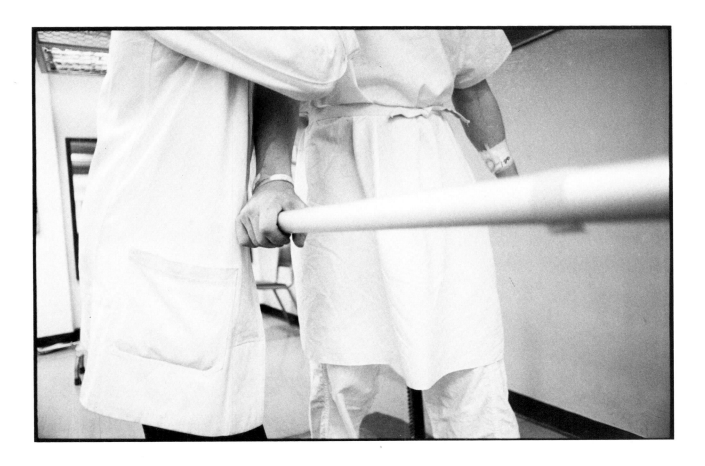

JOEL BRUINOOGE:
*Everything is so slow. What should take me a couple of seconds takes an hour. It's hard to do little things like go to the bathroom, or tie my shoe. Now these little things are big things.*

January 26, 1977

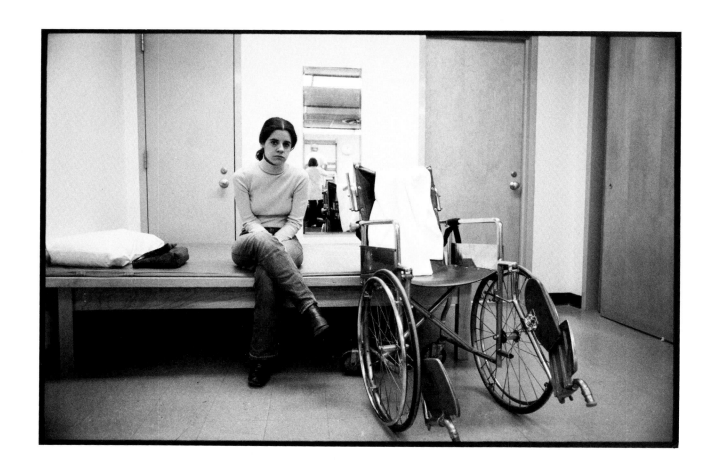

MEG CRISSARA:

*I remember the first time the physical therapist came in to try to help him walk. She picked him up but he wasn't doing very well and he couldn't take a step. I started to cry, and left the room so he wouldn't see.*

May 7, 1979

JOEL BRUINOOGE:
*This is not like anything else. I have never been in a place that I couldn't get out of. What scares me the most is the fear of being a cripple.*

January 26, 1977

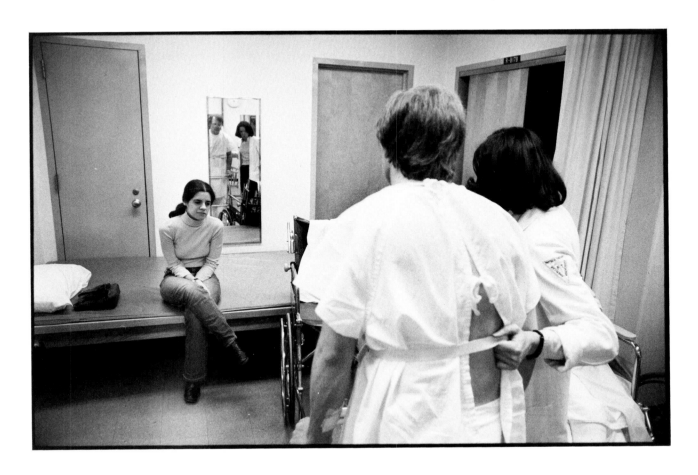

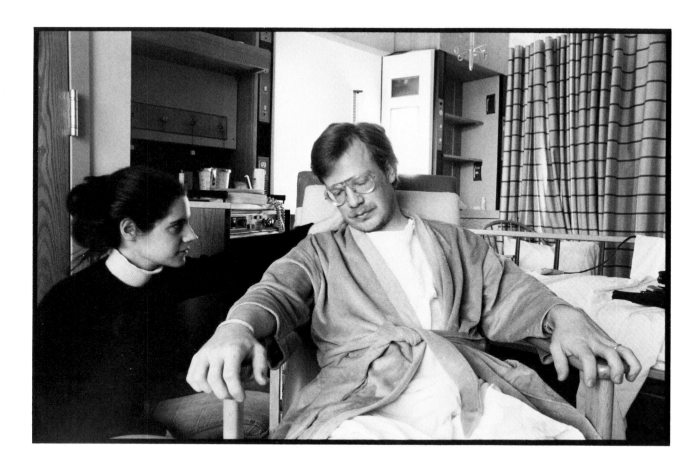

JOEL BRUINOOGE:

*Sometimes I start laughing like an idiot and can't stop. the part of my brain that was affected controlled my suppression reactions, so now things I would normally suppress automatically come to the surface. I feel like I don't have any control.*

MEG CRISSARA:

*I've loved you the whole time, but I like you even better now that you're so open about the way you feel. Sometimes, though, when I see a lot of laughing or crying I wonder whether you're actually feeling all that much...or whether your body's taking over.*

February 1, 1977

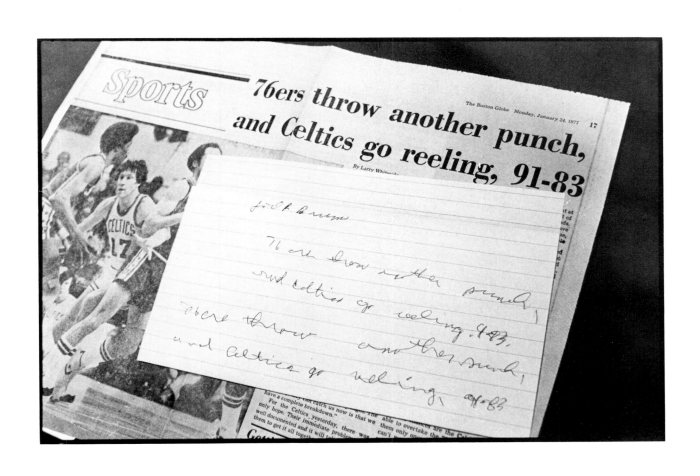

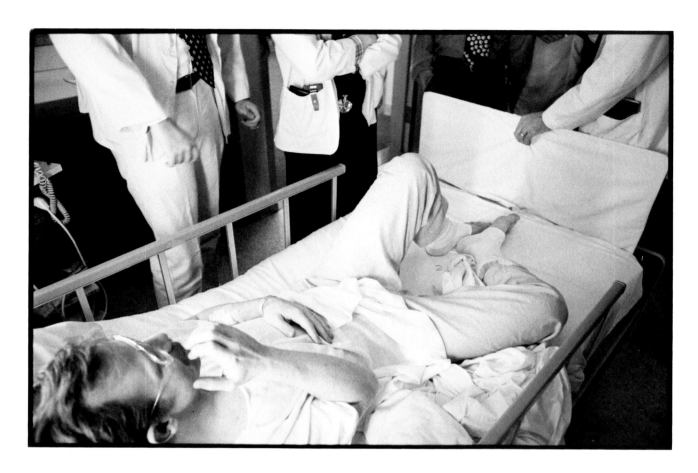

JOEL BRUINOOGE:
*It's funny to be a guinea pig for students. In the morning, all those people walk in and say, "Come on, do this, don't do that." It's like they're playing with me. "What's he gonna do today— jump hoops?"*

January 26, 1977

JON BRUINOOGE:
*Being able to help him with some of the physical things—like taking a shower, or wheeling him down to physical therapy— has made the waiting easier on us. I can also see changes on a day-to-day basis.*

*But Joel compares his abilities now with his abilities a month or six weeks ago, when he could do all kinds of things. A few days ago he felt that he was going to be home in a week and have no problems.*

January 26, 1977

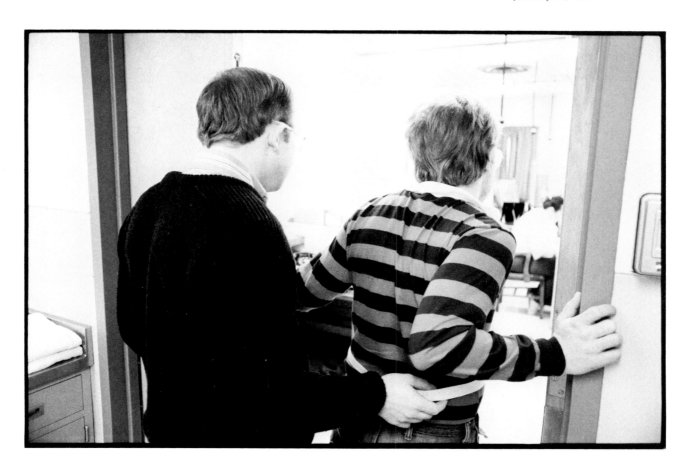

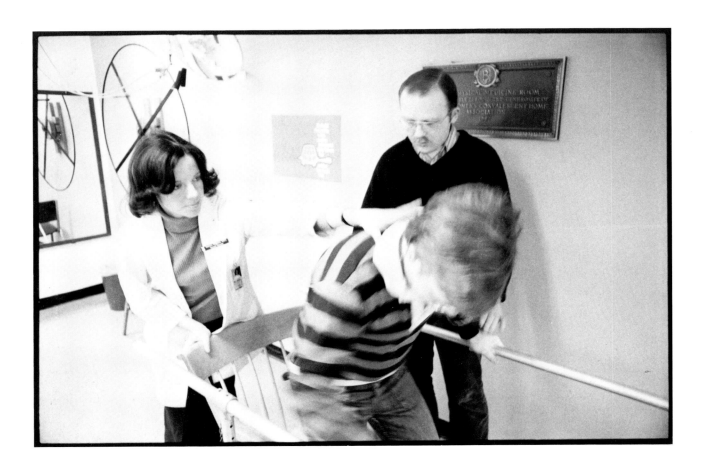

JOEL BRUINOOGE:
*Just today I got to the point where I could tell how well my balance was going. Before, I would be falling and I wouldn't know it; I couldn't tell what to do to stop it. It's a little bit frightening.*

February 1, 1977

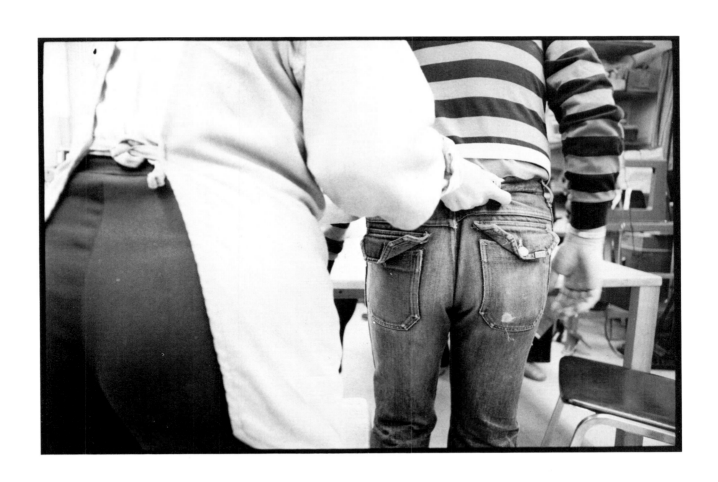

MEG CRISSARA:
(after Joel's return home)
*One of the basic areas where we communicated without having to talk was sex. It was always very nice and I never had to be the one that said, "Well, why don't we?" Now, we don't share that area of communication as often or as comfortably as before because it's a little bit awkward for him. He gets tired much faster. I don't walk around thinking about that but it's an outlet we just don't have now.*

April 7, 1977

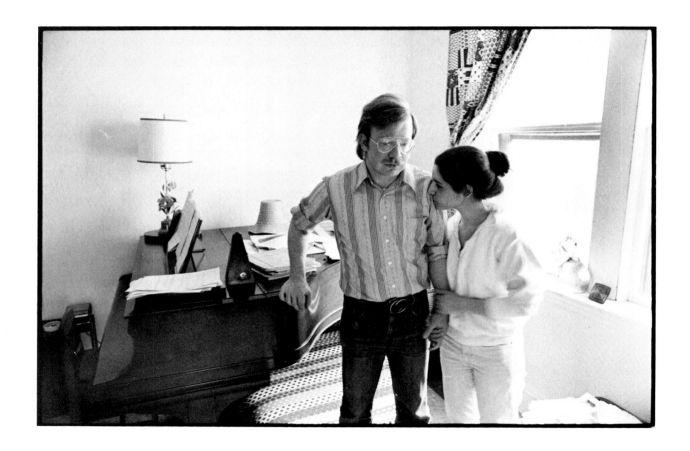

MEG CRISSARA:
*Sometimes Joel calls himself a cripple and I get absolutely un-done. We don't discuss it except to say, "Of course, everything's going to be fine," but underneath there is that big question.*

April 7, 1977

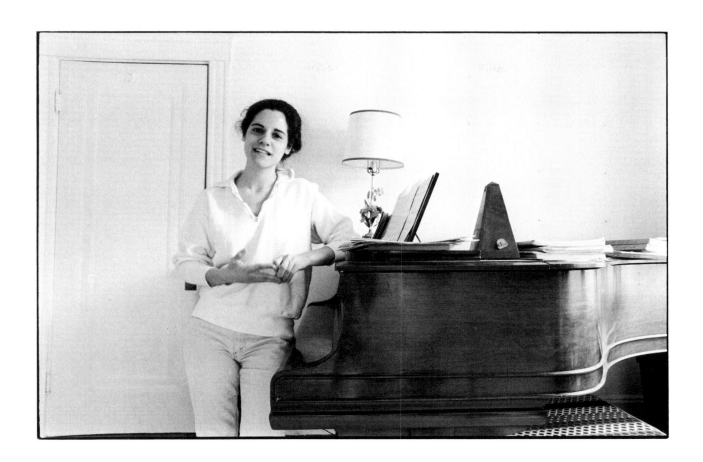

MEG CRISSARA:
*Joel had always been very supportive of me and, in a sense, our relationship centered around his doing as much as he could so I could practice the piano six hours a day and perform. When Joel was hospitalized, the rest of my life basically stopped.*

*All the stuff that we shared before is now my responsibility. Being emotionally strong and not falling apart is also my responsibility. If I'm home and I cry Joel asks me not to because it gets him upset. So I either have to go out to the sidewalk and cry, wait until he is out, or not cry at all.*

April 7, 1977

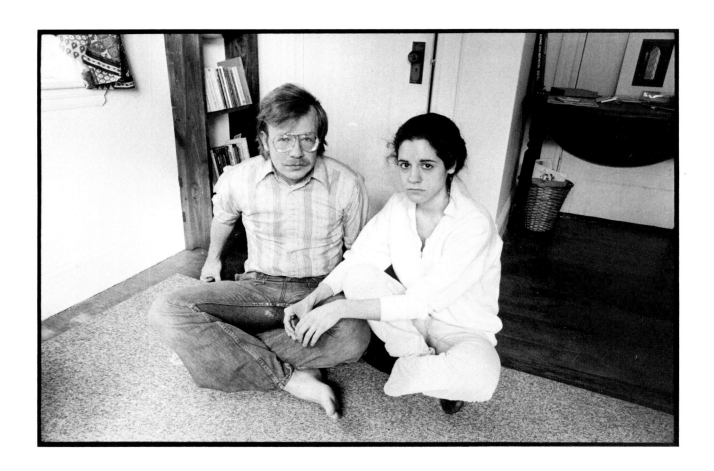

MEG CRISSARA:

*My friends and our parents are much more concerned about Joel than about me and that's understandable. If somebody calls and asks, "How are you doing," they really want to know how Joel is doing. Nobody says, "Well Meg, how are you?"*

*Joel used to ask, "What kind of a day did you have, what happened to you today?" He still does ask, but now he does it for form's sake—he's so busy getting better and the daily pressures on him are so incredible, that he can't really deal with my day.*

*I never had to give like this before. In the beginning I felt really great, my insides really wanted to give and when I found an outlet for it it really felt good. But now this has been going on long enough. It gets to be a strain.*

April 7, 1977

JOEL BRUINOOGE:
*I could tell you that it's very frustrating to try to learn how to tie your shoes for the first time, or it's very frustrating to have your attention span be only five minutes, but I don't think you would appreciate that unless you had gone through it, or you had seen someone you knew well have to struggle with it.*

January 1, 1979

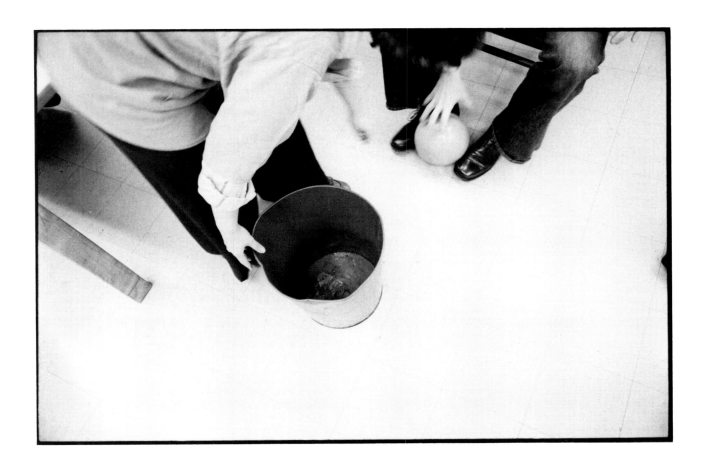

MEG CRISSARA:

*Those of our friends who have been through either a death or serious sickness in their family are immediately much more sensitive to our situation. They understand many things that our other friends just don't. Some people think it's not so hard because the changes in Joel are not so dramatic. Actually this is much harder than if Joel had had surgery or had been very sick and then gotten much better. This is harder—it takes more patience.*

March 6, 1977

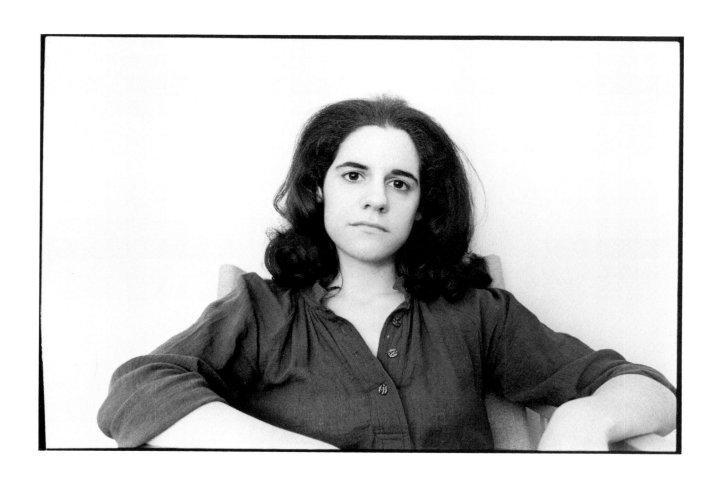

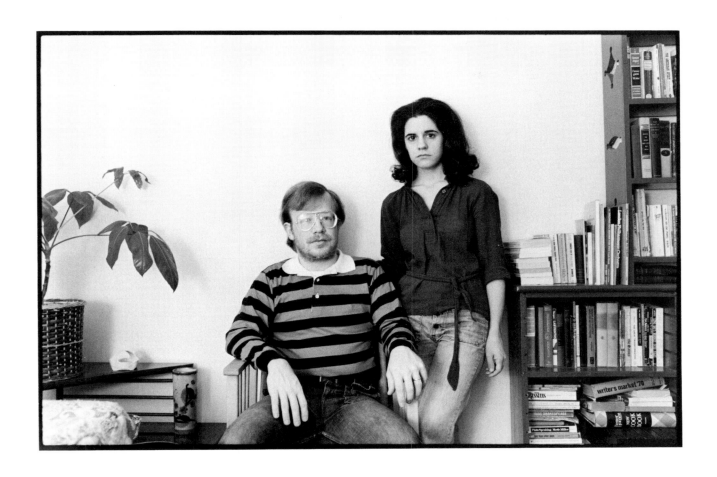

MEG CRISSARA:
*Even when people who are close to us call up wanting to see how we are, they will never refer to what actually happened to Joel nor ask him how he really is. They always say, "Gee, you look fine, ya know. Everything's gonna be all right." They're embarrassed, but they keep it all underneath: they know something's funny, Joel knows something's funny, but nobody will say anything about it.*

March 6, 1977

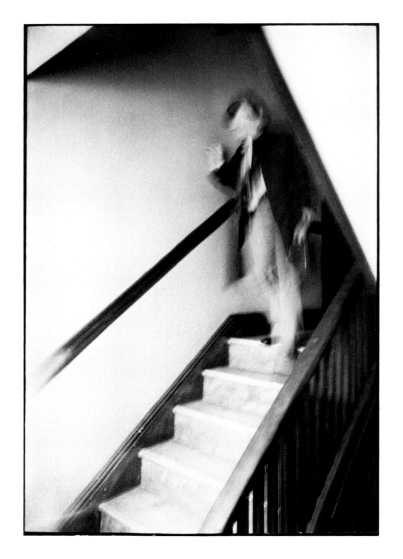

JOEL BRUINOOGE:

*The neurological damage makes me look like I'm drunk, and
every time I have to move I can see people say, "Hey, what's
with him?" It also means an incredible amount of work to stand
up on the subway all the way to downtown. I tried carrying a
cane so people would give me a seat. I ended up standing,
holding the cane.*

MEG CRISSARA:

*Since Joel talks a little slower and not quite as loudly as he used
to everybody talks more slowly and louder to him. His slow
speech makes it sound like his mind isn't working either. People
can't separate what comes out of his mouth from what's going
on in his head. It's like seeing a blind person and assuming he is
deaf as well as blind.*

JOEL BRUINOOGE:

*It's like I'm some kind of dummy.*                March 6, 1977

MEG CRISSARA:

*At the hospital Joel was getting a lot of encouragement and feedback every day about how well he was doing. It means a lot more to be told by a therapist or a doctor that you're getting better than if your wife just says, "Gee, you look better today." So today we went back to the hospital for therapy, and everyone who means something to Joel medically told him he was much better.*

February 13, 1977

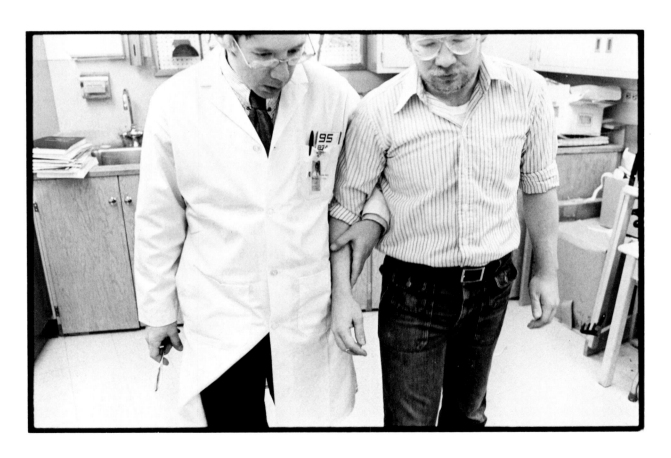

JOEL BRUINOOGE:

*I'm kind of stuck where I am. I will probably spend the rest of my working life with the same employer because, obviously, another company is not going to want to assume my medical risk—it's just easier to get somebody who doesn't have these problems. Freelance writing is out now, because I need the medical benefits I get with my job and I can't buy them on the open market.*

MEG CRISSARA:

*When Joel went back to work a week ago, they gave him a physical exam. They asked him to count backwards from one hundred by threes and he started to do it faster than the nurse could figure out if he was correct or not. I think it was like being insulted to be asked these things. Joel also had to get completely undressed then dressed again within less than an hour-and-a-half—a big, huge effort. That physical exam was so painful that Joel cried the whole afternoon and evening—it took a full day before he could even say what was bothering him.*

JOEL BRUINOOGE:

*It made me feel like a turkey because they wanted to see if I could think or not.*

September 11, 1977

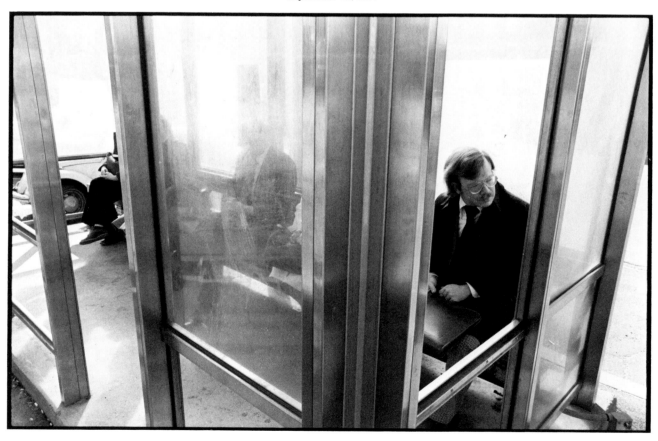

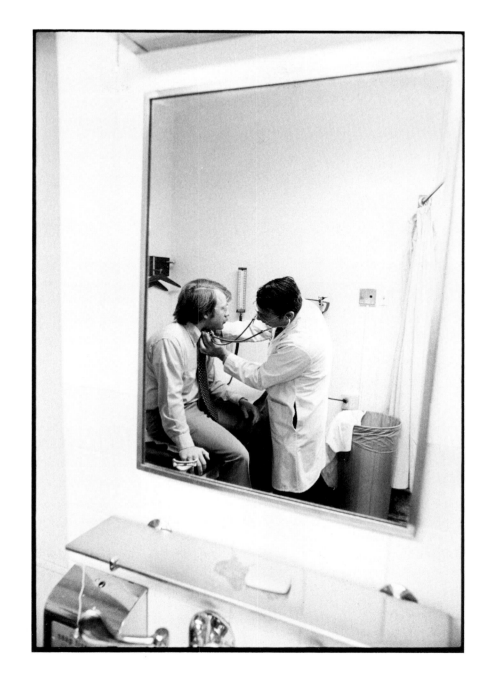

JOEL BRUINOOGE:

*Dr. Caplan stood out as a very human, compassionate person.
The biggest thing on my mind at that time was the financial
pressure from $20,000 of medical bills and my inability to work.
Caplan just said "look, if the insurance doesn't cover anything,
we'll just forget about it." He also called me one day at work, just
to see how I was.*

February 20, 1978

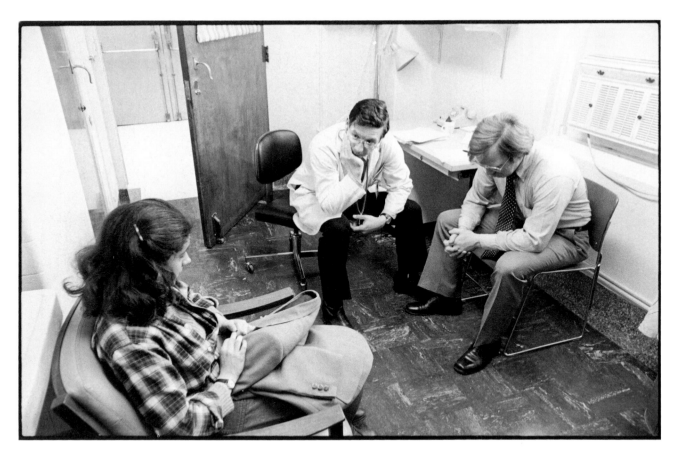

MEG CRISSARA:

*I don't think anybody should have told us any more or any less than they did, but at that time it was very frustrating. My greatest concern was how much is Joel going to recover and they would say, "He's doing very well," or "We think there's going to be a lot of recovery," and I'd say, "How much recovery?" At one point they said, "Well, we're going to expect at least eighty percent." But eighty percent doesn't mean anything if you don't know what the other twenty percent is going to be. Those numbers are really a trap.*

April 7, 1977

MEG CRISSARA:

*In the midst of being an extraordinarily busy man, Dr. Caplan never seemed hurried. When he was with Joel, I got the feeling that was all that was on his mind. Even two years after his stroke, Joel still felt so strongly about him that when he found out Dr. Caplan was moving to Chicago, he wrote him a note: "I'll have to be careful to have any more neurological problems in Chicago. Good luck to you." That was a very uncharacteristic thing for Joel to do. He felt so sad. It's a relationship that is very intimate, but then it's over quickly and completely.*

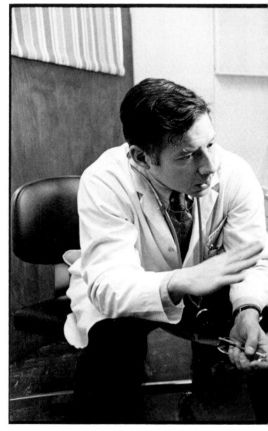

May 9, 1979

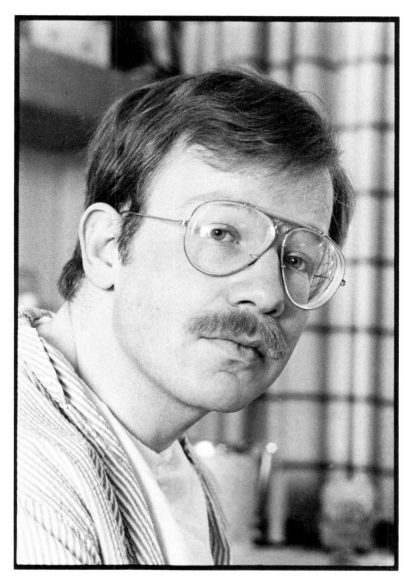

JOEL BRUINOOGE:

*On April 21st, about ten o'clock, I just had a little bit of chest pain. I had had pain like that before but the doctor had thought it was caused just by anxiety. I thought I'd go to sleep and it would go away. It was still there in the morning when I woke up, so I got dressed and took the subway to work. It hurt pretty bad and I started to perspire on the subway. It started to hurt worse at work so I went to the clinic and they sent me here. When I got here they gave me morphine and said I was having a heart attack.*

May 10, 1977

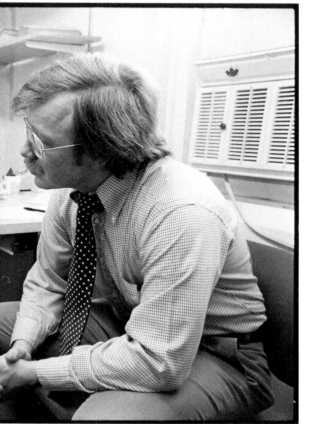

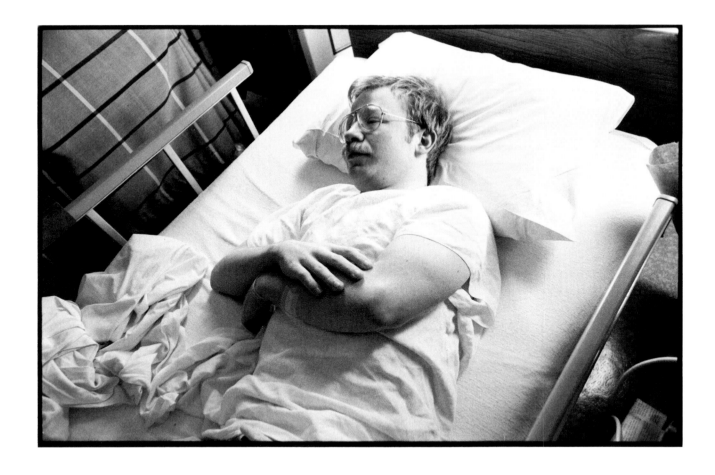

JOEL BRUINOOGE:

*I remember lying in the hospital bed after the heart attack think-ing that my problems now had become very finite: whether I could move my left hand or whether I could pick up that nickel. It was a relief. I had the very strong feeling that the lifestyle I had been living was wrong for me—for example instead of doing what I wanted to do I would end up carting Meg around so she could do what she wanted to do: play a concert or practice. The stroke and the heart attack gave me a chance to say I quit, they were a way out.*

May 7, 1979

JOEL BRUINOOGE:

*Medical students just come in and expect you to do something when and because they want you to do it. During breakfast you just have to stop eating to be examined. They never stop to ask what I'll be doing or set up a particular time to come by. They say they'll call back...but they don't, like they think it doesn't make any difference. My intern comes in at weird hours like ten or eleven o'clock at night. She seems more concerned about what other people are going to think of her than she is concerned about what is good for me.*

May 10, 1977

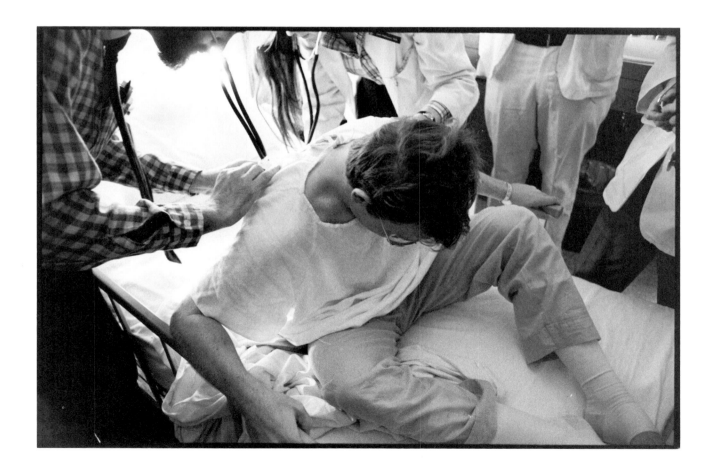

MEG CRISSARA:

*We were very normal, but what that experience does to normal people is profound, and confusing, and very, very frightening. There was Joel, this sick person, in a place that is technologically as sophisticated as anywhere in the world, and in all the time he was there no one came by to see if he was depressed or wanting to talk to someone about how he felt. I wasn't even told you could ask to have somebody come by. Maybe our appearance of being strong hid the fact that we needed help.*

May 9, 1979

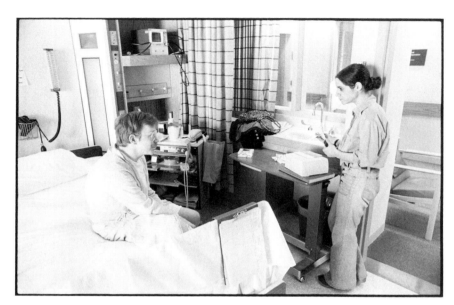

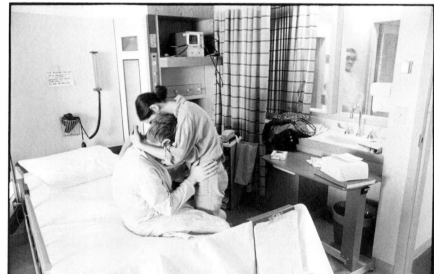

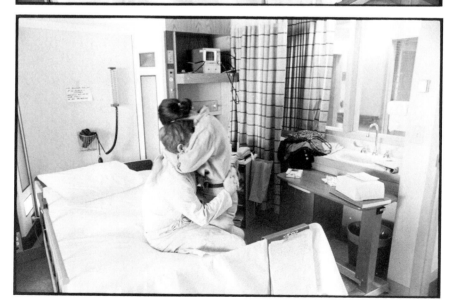

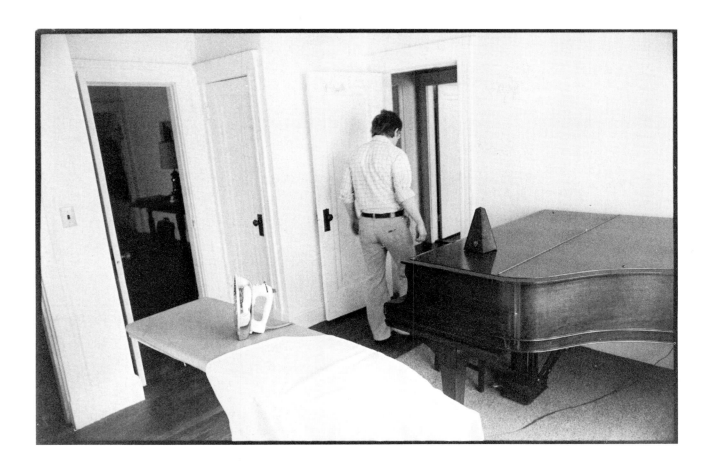

JOEL BRUINOOGE:

*Meg said she wanted to separate the day I came home from the hospital after the heart attack. I think even before I had had the stroke there were tensions in the marriage. I was more pragmatic than she was—because I had to be. I felt I had assumed more than my share of housekeeping and domestic responsibilities. I took care of everything and she concentrated her total awareness on playing the piano. She was not interested in my job—she wanted me to quit and write a novel— and I wanted her to pursue a career with financial rewards.*

*My illness brought these differences to a head. It threw the total load of daily chores—from buying food to making out the income tax—on her. It forced a complete change in her life's priorities, and she was afraid it would limit what she was going to do with her piano. It was life-threatening in a sense: it threatened our hopes of what our lives were going to be.*

September 11, 1977

JOEL BRUINOOGE:

*Meg left about two weeks after I came home from the hospital. She felt that the stroke and the heart attack were harder on her than on me. At first I was pretty angry. I felt betrayed. Then the anger was replaced by a sense of loneliness.*

*I haven't told people at work because I don't want to demonstrate any sign of instability. My doctors haven't asked about it. They say, "Give my regards to Meg." and I just go, "Sure," because I don't want the hassle of having to explain.*

September 11, 1977

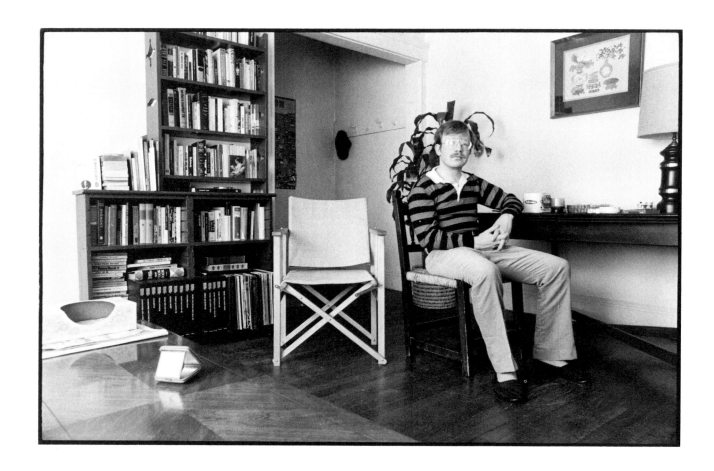

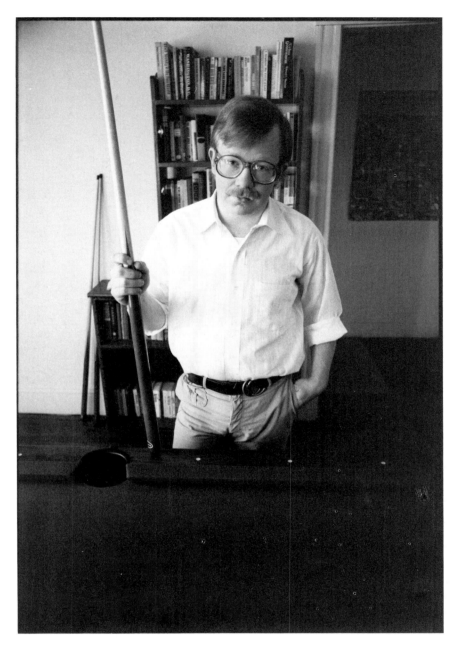

JOEL BRUINOOGE:

*After the heart attack, the cardiologist told Meg I could probably never be a father because the strain of staying up all night or playing with kids would be too much. He wouldn't talk to me about it because he felt it would be unwise to subject a patient to the stress that kind of discussion would generate.*

*But the real stress for me was living in dread that something else was going to happen. I don't know any better now whether I'll have another heart attack or stroke, but I can't go through my life waiting for it to happen.*

September 11, 1977

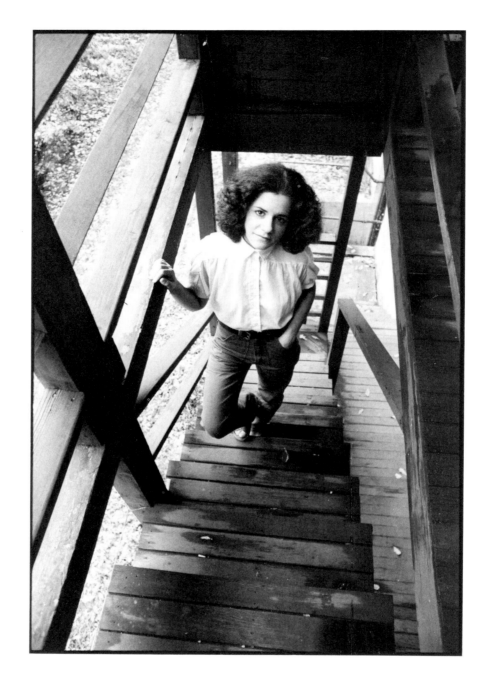

MEG CRISSARA:
*After Joel began to recover, his feeling was, "Oh, I can live, I can, oh, wow, how great! I can go back to work! Look at this, I can get dressed!" My feeling was, please, I need to rest.*

*I needed to take time for those things that don't count in terms of dollars or cents or getting ahead. There are more important things to do than worry all the time—and in our marriage there was an awful lot of worry an awful lot of the time.*

May 9, 1979

MEG CRISSARA:

*We were both pushed to the brink and made to question what it means to be living. But after stepping away from that, the quality of day-to-day life just changes; it's just much, much fuller. Still if someone had suggested to me while I was going through it, that it was going to be a positive experience, I probably would have told them to shut the hell up. I didn't want to hear it.*

*If I was around somebody going through the same thing now, I would probably be real quiet, and try to just be there, just listen, and take the person out for dinner. Get them out of the hospital for a little while, take them for a walk. That help is even more necessary after the tension and trauma are over, once the person is back home.*

May 9, 1979

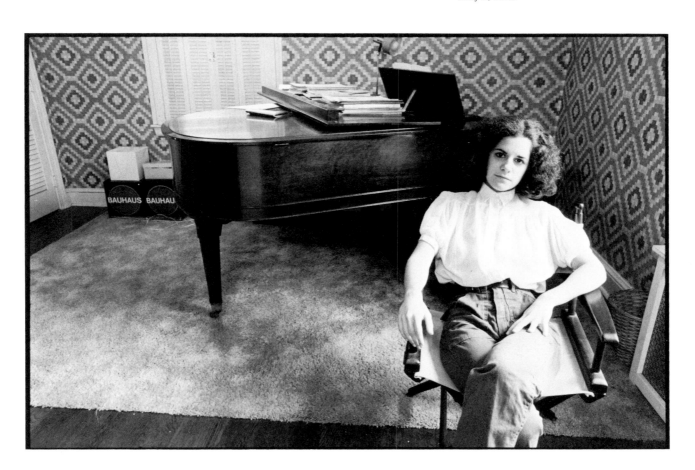

JOEL BRUINOOGE:

*In some ways I consider myself very lucky for having had the experience. It's allowed me a chance to sit back and look at my life. I'm happier with the way I live now than I was before I had the stroke.*

*After I had the stroke I decided that I didn't want to expend energy on playing games with people, telling them what they want to hear. It's not just being more honest with myself—it's being more honest with other people.*

*Work is less stressful because I can look at situations that would have produced stress for me before and say, "That's not a problem—I have had problems."*

May 7, 1979

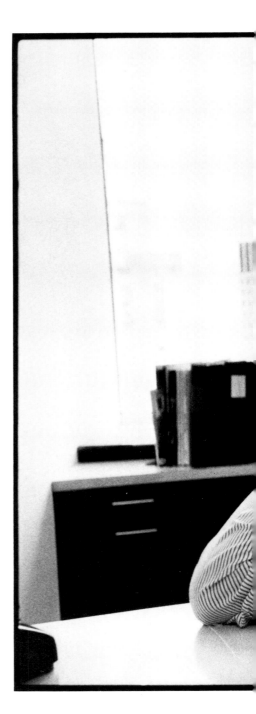

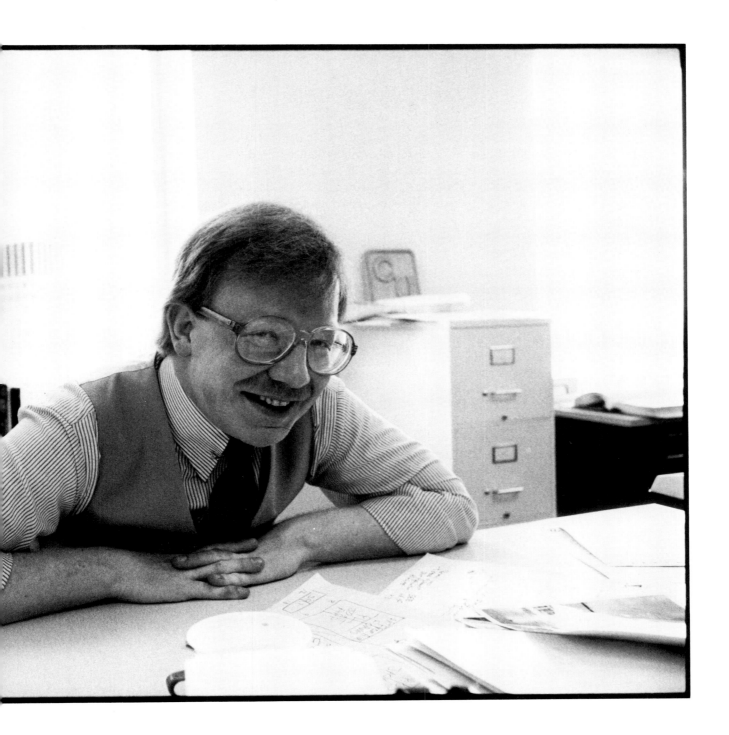

# A Perspective on Patients
## by Mark L. Rosenberg, M.D.

This section relates the subjective experiences of these six patients to some general observations on illness and health care. Many of these observations come from the work of medical sociologists who try to understand how people behave in particular roles and settings. Their studies have focused on the roles of patient and physician. The short bibliography at the end of this section will introduce the reader to some of the literature from which much of this discussion derives.

### From Person to Patient

People do not think of themselves as patients when they feel well. Even when they have a physical problem, they often choose to live with it for a while, hoping that it will go away on its own, or hoping they might get better with a home remedy or with the advice of a friend or newspaper article. Surveys of large groups of people have shown that at any one time, up to 92 percent of the population have ailments that could be diagnosed and/or treated by a physician, but only a very small fraction of those people seek a doctor's care.

People react to their symptoms differently, and their reactions may be explained in part by their backgrounds and past experiences. Some people feel that certain aches and pains are just a part of life, a hazard of the job, or part of growing old; in any case, something one has to put up with. Specific cultural factors such as ethnic background or socioeconomic status may affect the way an individual experiences a particular physical change. One author concerned with the perception of pain found that within his study population, Italians tended to focus on the immediate pain associated with a particular ailment; their primary concern was pain relief. Jewish subjects thought their pain meant that their bodies were falling apart, and did not mind the pain as much as they feared its implications. Irish subjects tended to accept pain as part of life, denying that anything was really wrong. Kay Finn's Irish background offers one possible explanation for why she lived with pain in her breast and pain in her back for almost a year before she sought medical attention.

One can imagine several additional reasons why Kay Finn might have delayed in seeking medical care. She said that she did not want to think of herself as a patient, because to her, patients were old people who were dependent on doctors, drugs, and canes, and she valued her independence. She was afraid of what she might be told. She didn't want to go to the hospital alone; perhaps she did not want to be left alone. In addition, she did not understand that the pain in her back represented the spread of cancer to her spine; she did not even know that cancer could spread like that. Jeanne McLaughlin delayed for different reasons. She felt that her husband was too ill to be left alone when she first discovered the lump in her breast—at least that was her stated reason; she may have had others. Jenny Monroe's mother had noticed that Jenny's eye turned in, but she thought that she was the only person who had noticed it, and she hoped it would correct itself.

Illness may be so sudden and so severe that it cannot be denied, but even under these circumstances, the individual may delay in seeking care. When he had his first heart attack, Ed MacPhee had such bad chest pain that he had to lie down on the couch; he was unable to get his breath and was sick to his stomach. But he waited until this recurred before he went to the hospital. A few years later, he fainted at the subway station and was rushed to the hospital by ambulance. Joel Bruinooge had mild symptoms early in the day and attributed his dizziness to fatigue. But he sought medical attention quickly when he found himself unable to walk or talk. Although early medical intervention cannot always prevent or minimize the consequences of a disease, it is clear that people sometimes delay too long in seeking medical care because their judgment is impaired. At those times, friends and family can provide important counsel and support.

People may also delay in seeking care because they cannot pay for care, because they believe the symptom or disease is not serious or they are invulnerable, or because they feel that nothing can be done for them. Additioinal barriers to obtaining care might include inaccessibility, lack of transportation, lack of child care, or lack of a vocabulary through which to articulate one's concern.

## Aspects of the Patient Role

The individual who has made the transition from healthy person to patient may find that those around him—both physicians and nonphysicians—expect him to act in particular ways: he should want to get better, he should do what he is told by the doctor, and in return, he is exempted from certain obligations, such as his usual work or family duties. Ed MacPhee welcomed the chance to sit back and take orders, and parlayed his exemption from work and family duties into a retirement lifestyle of almost exclusively leisure pursuits. Sandy Heywood, however, was eager to escape from a state of potentially permanent patienthood, and resented people telling her she should not go to school or work because she was a dialysis patient.

In the beginning, some people may blame themselves for their illnesses. They might feel that if they had acted differently or had sought care sooner, they might have avoided the disease or its complications. This may reflect in part our need to find a reason for everything. The recent emphasis on personal responsibility for one's health, stressing preventive measures and healthy lifestyles, may increase the individual's tendency to blame himself for his illness, especially for diseases like cancer whose causes are not understood. Self-blame may defeat an effective attempt at recovery. In addition, the patient may pick up cues that other people blame him or her for all or part of the illness. Kay Finn probably learned from the unsubtle questioning of some physicians she saw when she was hospitalized that she had been "stupid and careless" in letting her illness go for so long before seeking care. Sandy Heywood felt that she might have caused her illness by taking excessive quantities of aspirin, although none of her doctors could have known that.

Pain is a common accompaniment of illness. It can color the patient's whole life, and make even the simplest task an awesome and grueling experience. Kay Finn's movements in bed were so excruciating that even getting an X-ray became an ordeal. Individuals may experience the pain associated with a physical state or procedure differently, depending on what the pain signifies to them. During World War II, for example, soldiers who had received severe injuries, such as traumatic amputation of a leg, required almost no anesthetic at all if they interpreted their injury as a ticket home from the war. On the other hand, Kay Finn's pain may have been particularly severe for her since she knew it came from the cancer that would ultimately kill her.

It may also be more difficult for friends and family to sympathize with an individual in pain when its causes are not visible. Ed MacPhee found that friends could not understand why his angina kept him from keeping pace with their walking and talking. Indeed, to avoid lengthy explanations of his illness, he started avoiding his friends altogether. Fatigue presents a similar problem in many respects. Sandy Heywood may not look any different when she has just completed dialysis and her blood count is low, but she may feel exhausted and might remain fatigued throughout the next day. Most of us have been tired and have been in pain, but it is hard to remember just what we felt like at those times. While this has an adaptive benefit for us—making our memories and lives generally more pleasant—it also makes it harder to empathize with the patient.

Coping with pain and fatigue takes many forms. Ed MacPhee retired from work, slowed down his general pace, and stopped to take nitroglycerin when he needed it. Sandy Heywood adjusted her lifestyle so that on days following dialysis treatments, she could keep her activities at a minimum. Joel Bruinooge slowed his pace and found that he was able to relax as he never had before. Aids to coping with pain come in the form of drugs—often with the side effect of making the patient drowsy or dopey—surgical procedures, meditation, hypnosis, and counseling. The changes in the person's lifestyle necessitated by pain or fatigue may impose hardships on the patient's family who now must assume roles and do chores formerly managed by the patient.

Illness can be stigmatizing, imposing additional burdens upon the patient. Although contagion is now rarely a real issue, patients may become psychologically isolated because family or friends harbor fears about the illness. This is particularly true for diseases that are poorly understood. Again, cancer is a clear example. The word cancer means crab, a slow, silent, sinister beast that consumes its victim—an image strong enough to frighten most people. It is associated with ugliness, and this association, together with the frightening likelihood that this poorly understood illness attacks indiscriminately, can lead friends and family to establish a distance between themselves and the patient. Sandy Heywood wondered about herself after her kidneys had been removed. Was she "some kind of freak who had no kidneys and couldn't pee?" Meg Crissara found friends talking around the issues, unable to discuss Joel's illness with her directly.

Mental illness carries even greater stigmata, perhaps because of some of the same ungrounded fears of contagion. With these stigmata in mind, in relating his history to his cardiac surgeon, Ed MacPhee omitted his experiences with alcoholism and a nervous breakdown. And when he was hospitalized on the psychiatric ward of the Veterans Hospital, he was reluctant to tell anyone other than his wife. Part of the stigmatizing effect of illness is fear of the unknown; familiarity with the illness might diminish that fear, allowing family and friends to approach the patient more closely, to accompany him when he needs their support.

Acceptance of illness means more than accepting one's physical limitations, pain, and fatigue. It means thinking about how the illness may change one's future, one's work and ability to earn an income, and one's ability to discharge family responsibilities. The changes that illness effects can pervade a person's entire existence. An illness may serve as a focal point around which one's life may be reorganized. For Joel Bruinooge, it led to major changes in the way he related to his wife and his work. His illness meant that initially Meg had to perform all the routine household tasks. This led to resentment on her part and guilt on Joel's part. They had to examine their relationship; their long-term accommodation involved a separation with increased independence for both people.

If we fall into the trap of thinking that the patient restricts his concerns about his illness to those times when we discuss the illness with him, we may underestimate the disturbance that a serious illness can create and in turn underestimate the patient's need for support. This is particularly likely to happen when patients try to appear strong, as did Meg and Joel, or when they try to appear independent. "I was looking for company badly," Kay Finn said, "but I don't think the people I was talking to realized how badly I was wanting company. Because I tried to act so independent, and underneath it all, I'm not. I'm human, that's all."

Because of anxieties, both in the patient and in the family, communication between the patient and others frequently breaks down just when all involved are most in need of support. The patient may need to be supported in acknowledging his own fears, anxiety, and sadness in facing the threat of loss that his illness poses, whether it be a short-term loss of strength or time from work, or a permanent loss of a body part or function. Some patients may deny part of their illness and choose to avoid talking about it for a while, but this doesn't mean they are unaware of it. More frequently, they may search for a sign of interest from family or friend, a signal that the friend is willing to listen to them and look at them. Listening and understanding are valuable and supportive in themselves, and should not be confused with pity. A patient's fear that revealing his illness may evoke pity or fear from a friend can lead him to avoid mentioning it. This can create the disturbing situation in which patient and friend sit in silence, each having the illness uppermost in his mind, aware that the other knows, and using all their mental energies to avoid discussing what concerns them both most. In a similar way, when a family member is afraid to mention his concerns to the patient—concerns that the patient may very well share—he may foster a frustrating and distancing silence.

Communication occurs in many forms. A large part of the ordinary communication between husband and wife, for example, may be indirect. Joel Bruinooge's illness led to a temporary cessation of sexual intercourse with his wife, Meg. This activity had been very important for both of them as a form of nonverbal communication. Jeanne McLaughlin's husband refused to sleep in bed with her after her mastectomy. Although he said he was afraid of hurting her in the area of her recent surgery, she felt he avoided her because he did not want to look at her scar. His behavior communicated rejection.

The patient's fear that "everyone already knows" may also make it difficult for the patient to talk to people with whom he or she prefers not to discuss the illness. It was not until several months after returning to work that Jeanne McLaughlin, wearing a breast prosthesis and clothes that fit well, realized that not everyone who saw her could know she had had a mastectomy. Sometimes, however, a change is apparent and an illness cannot be hidden or denied. Jenny Monroe's friends could see she wore glasses, and they asked her quite directly, "Why?" and just as directly, she told them, "Because my eye is crooked." Being asked why didn't disturb her; not being asked and being called "four-eyes" did. Joel Bruinooge also found he could not conceal his illness. Although his gait and speech disturbances were obvious, he found that when some of his co-workers had difficulty understanding him, they felt it impolite to ask him to repeat himself. Since his job as public relations director depended on clear communications, he found it most helpful to begin interviews by asking people to let him know if they had difficulty understanding what he said, and by acknowledging that he had a speech defect due to a stroke. A straightforward statement, he felt, would clear the air and was essential to effective communication.

## Patients in the Hospital

The hospital environment may have a tremendous effect on how the patient feels. Nowhere else are people so clearly identified as either patients or nonpatients. Patients have hospital numbers, gowns, beds, charts, pills, and operations; hospital staff workers and visitors do not. And additional differences—not necessarily real ones—may be perceived by the patients.

They have illnesses, nonpatients do not; they have problems, nonpatients do not; they've lost their identifying surroundings, clothes, and positions; and perhaps most important, in part by being identified as patients, they've lost their sense of well-being.

Entry into the hospital often marks a shift from the vertical to the horizontal position, which itself can have profound psychological effects. Kay Finn spent hours lying down—waiting on a stretcher in a hallway, waiting to be taken to or from the radiology department. Even a healthy individual who is made to disrobe and lie down feels defenseless and despondent. When that person is ill, psychologically dependent on doctors and nurses, and physically dependent on someone to push his stretcher or wheelchair, he may feel totally helpless. Once in the hospital, Kay Finn felt entirely dependent on doctors and nurses: "At this point," she said, "who else can do for you?"

Even those patients who are able to walk unassisted are frequently not allowed to travel within the hospital on their own. Instead, they are transported in beds or wheelchairs. This loss of mobility can be frustrating and demoralizing.

Hospital procedures and schedules confine a patient to his room so that he can be available when staff members visit to interview, examine, diagnose, or treat him. Schedules for meals and sleep are determined by, and for the convenience of, hospital workers, rather than patients. Before Joel went into the hospital, he scheduled his own appointments and controlled his own time. In the hospital, it was very different. Not only did the many health care workers who came to see him not come by appointment, but they often came at times that were particularly inconvenient or times when he had visitors. The busy schedules of his physicians and the demands of hospital scheduling increased Joel's sense of loss of control at a time when he was struggling to regain physical control of his body.

The physical limitations imposed by illness don't end once the patient leaves the hospital. Jeanne McLaughlin was out of work for six weeks after her mastectomy, a long time for the family who depended on her work for financial support. Kay Finn's back pain made her give up her daily walks. To her, dependence on a cane signaled old age and the end of her life. When Joel first left the hospital, it took him an hour to get dressed, and because of his balance and gait disturbance, he could not ride the subway to work on his previous schedule because he feared being pushed over by the press of the crowds. At the same time, his restricted diet—no cholesterol, no sugar, no salt, no alcohol, no smoking—seemed to him to limit his ability to socialize, eat, and drink with friends. Ed MacPhee's daily life had been scheduled around the frequent times he had to take his medications—he used to set an alarm clock to wake up to take his night-time doses. Even after surgery, he felt his life depended on medicines. Sandy Heywood spends five hours a day, three days a week, on the dialysis machine and additional time commuting to the Kidney Center. Without dialysis, she would die. Sandy's clear dependence on the dialysis machine made it very important for her to establish and maintain her independence in other aspects of her life. It was important for her to have her own apartment and she chose not to consider home dialysis—where the cleansing of her blood would be done in her own home—because she did not want the dialysis equipment in her apartment as a constant reminder of her dependence. With the help of her physician, she arranged to be dialyzed at facilities in other parts of the country so she could get away for vacations.

The costs of acute or chronic illness often make patients financially dependent as well. This burden falls most heavily on individuals who are not covered by health insurance, the "medically indigent," who have too much money to qualify for government assistance and not enough to buy private health insurance. The six patients we've seen were lucky to have had some form of health insurance to cover their health care costs. Ed MacPhee's surgery and ten-day hospitalization, for example, cost more than $10,000. But even with her health care costs covered, Sandy Heywood found it very difficult to achieve financial independence. She was unable to accept an offer for a $10,000 per year job because she would have lost more than $12,000 a year in government-paid health and welfare benefits.

### Leaving the Patient Role

While the initial phase of a severe illness can be devastating in its abruptness, later phases can be equally or even more stressful if they present the patient with a permanent disability or the specter of a progressively downhill course. Once the initial shock wears off, the patient must begin to readjust his or her life to accommodate the illness, and this period is fraught with its own difficulties. The transition from hospitalized patient back to the role of participant in family and work can be extremely stressful for all concerned. In the hospital, the patient was frequently the center of attention, his status was special, and he had a purpose and a goal—to get well and leave the hospital. But once he has left the hospital, he may feel abandoned, like Jeanne McLaughlin, or discouraged by the relative lack of attention he receives. The hard work of recovery may need to be carried on without help from this point, and this can be a slow and depressing process. As Ed MacPhee found, fatigue and weakness may persist for weeks or even months after the physical scars have healed. For some patients like Joel, returning to work is a tremendously important step, marking the final phase of the transition from patient back to person. Sandy Heywood, however, remained a "patient" even after she left the hospital and returned to school. Dependent on dialysis, she remained neither sick nor fully well, caught in the margin between the two states. How should she be viewed and treated by others? The least welcome alternative from her point of view was to be avoided by people who shared treating her inappropriately, as totally ill or totally well.

Some patients have no real chance of recovery and they must confront the prospect of their own death. It is important to realize that people may vary as much in the approaches they take to dying as they vary in their approaches to living. Kay Finn chose to deny that she was dying in the same way she had chosen to deny the seriousness of her illness. And Jeanne McLaughlin thought her husband wanted to deny that he was dying of cancer. It is difficult to judge just what, when, and how patients with terminal illnesses should be told. It is clearly tragic, however, if dying patients are isolated and abandoned when they most need support.

They frequently need physical as well as emotional support. Pain must be relieved and additional comforts provided. There is a growing interest now in efforts to provide special services for dying patients, either in their own homes or in the comfortable surroundings of a hospice. Either of these settings may be less alienating and discomforting than the technologically oriented acute-care hospital. When Kay Finn knew she was dying, she wanted to go home, but her repeated requests were interpreted by a physician as showing that she had "absolutely no insight into her condition." It was the physician who lacked insight. He thought patients went home only if they were improving, not to die. About one month before her death, Kay Finn continued the retreat that had begun with her hospitalization. She did not want any more photographs taken or discussions recorded. She did not want any visitors other than her sister. This progressive withdrawal was for her, as it is for many patients, part of her preparation for death.

### The Family

A patient's illness can affect everyone around him, and the greatest effect may be on those closest to him. The illness may necessitate a change in the usual family roles, as when a former breadwinner is no longer able to work and the spouse must assume responsibility for earning an income. Meg Crissara's primary occupation before Joel's illness was playing the piano; after Joel became ill, her new responsibilities left her little time to practice or perform. A parent's illness may mean he can no longer care for his children, but now must be cared for. Whether these changes are permanent or temporary, they can be very difficult. When Kay Finn was bedridden at home, her sister assumed the new role of nurse. As difficult as it was for Mrs. McCarthy physically at age 70, it was even more difficult emotionally to see and feel responsible for her sister in pain. As a result, Kay Finn was hospitalized because there was no one to take care of her at home, a situation that is becoming increasingly prevalent as the extended family becomes less common.

Illness can impose an additional financial stress on the family if a breadwinner loses time from work to stay home and care for the patient. And while health insurance frequently pays for most expenses incurred during a hospitalization, it almost never covers expenses incurred for home care.

### Health Care Personnel

Part of what makes the experience of illness difficult for both patients and families is the uncertainty concerning the outcome. As Meg Crissara said, that uncertainty was always in the air, and crossed her mind every ten minutes. In many cases, the outcome is no clearer to the physician, and his own uncertainty about disease and treatment outcomes may make him feel that he is equally uncertain about anything the patient would want to know. Dr. Monroe, for example, felt that patients craved information and that a physician could never tell them enough. If indeed what the patient craves is reassurance, then Dr. Monroe is correct in stating that no amount of technical information about the course of the disease will provide that reassurance. But physicians do know much about diseases and their treatments which they can share with patients and their families.

Traditionally little of this information has been passed on to patients. In part, this may relate to practices at a time when medicine lacked a broad scientific base and was largely a set of secret potions and black magic passed down with a professional code that forbade sharing those secrets with nonphysicians. The traditions surrounding the selection and training of native curers, healers, and witch doctors often serve a similar purpose—to maintain the status and power of the practitioner. Some contemporary sociologists argue that knowledge is power and that physicians maintain control over their patients by deliberately keeping their patients ignorant of "the medical facts." In some cases, physicians may feel they do not have enough time to explain to the patient what they view as overly involved technical details of an illness or its treatment. While it is true that it would be a time-consuming task to share with a patient everything the physician knows about the illness, it usually is not difficult to explain basic concepts clearly. In fact, in typical doctor-patient encounters in a primary care setting, physicians spend very little time on explanations of any sort. One investigator found that in visits that lasted an average of 20 minutes, the physician spent an average of only 1.2 minutes conveying information about an illness to the patient.

Irrespective of the reason, however, the amount of information many people possess about their own illnesses is frequently very small. Kay Finn, for example, did not know that cancer could spread to her bones. Perhaps, if she had known that, she would have sought medical attention sooner, when a surgical procedure still might have helped her.

Increased knowledge will not always result in a change in behavior, but information does sometimes have this effect. It has been shown, for example, that people are more likely to follow their physicians' suggestions when they understand why they are expected to do so. Other researchers have found that patients who had been told what to expect after surgery required less pain medication post-operatively. In any case, knowledge about one's illness may help a person feel more in control, less frightened, and better able to plan particular aspects of his or her own life. When Jeanne McLaughlin learned that she could make the choice between a radical and simple mastectomy, it was important for her to actually make that choice and assert control. Information about drug side effects could have alerted Ed MacPhee that the joint pains he developed probably resulted from one of his medications and should not have made him fear that he was developing yet another crippling illness. On the other hand, the relatively easy post-operative hospital courses of both Jenny Monroe and Ed MacPhee illustrate benefits of prior explanations in helping patients know what to expect.

These explanations need not be provided by the physician personally. A specially trained nurse-clinician met with Ed MacPhee for several hours both before and after his operation to discuss his surgery, the hospital routine during the post-operative period, and what he might expect after his discharge from the hospital. Printed information is also available in books, pamphlets, and articles published commercially and by disease-oriented associations such as the American Heart Association. Technical information as well as emotional support are frequently available from patients, former patients, and families who can be identified by health care personnel and who sometimes meet regularly as support and information-sharing groups. A rapidly increasing number of self-help and explanatory books by both physicians and lay people are also appearing. In addition, many patients may be able to use standard medical texts and journals as sources of information if they avoid overly technical articles and are willing to read with a medical dictionary in hand.

In some instances, patients may need to overcome the physicians' reluctance to present information they feel might be frightening to patients or their families. Jenny Monroe's mother was made anxious by Dr. Petersen's discussion of the risks of general anesthesia. In that case, recent legislation and legal decisions have made it clear that physicians have a legal responsibility to inform patients of the risks, benefits, and alternatives to surgical procedures. Dr. Petersen clearly recognized that this information would be disturbing to Mrs. Monroe, but believed he had no legal or ethical alternative. In the absence of legal requirements, however, many physicians will still choose to avoid presenting information they feel might arouse anxiety in the patient; instead, they choose to answer only those questions the patient asks. Whether or not this is the best solution to their dilemma, that choice suggests that the initiative for seeking information will frequently rest with the patient.

## Sharing Decision-Making Responsibility

It is difficult for most physicians to share decision-making responsibility with patients and their families. Even though her physician told her that the decision was hers, when Jeanne McLaughlin chose the simple mastectomy, her physician was angry enough to stand up and walk out on her. There are many possible explanations for the difficulty physicians might have in sharing decision-making responsibility with their patients. Some people argue that physicians are used to occupying a special status in our culture. Coming mostly from middle or upper-middle class backgrounds, their median income is higher than that of 95 percent of the population and the importance of their work is not to be questioned. They are "professionals" with an unusual degree of technical expertise whose role dictates that they put the interest of their clients before their own. Should they then have to answer to non-professionals who are motivated by self-interest?

The profession has tended to attract individuals who value independence and autonomy. their subsequent medical education stresses the importance of their assuming responsibility for their patients' well-being as well as the unique importance of clinical experience—which only medical education and practice can provide. How, they might then ask, could individuals without either this responsibility or experience be competent to make decisions about medical questions?

The nature of medical work tends to reinforce the physician's belief that he or she alone can make these decisions. One medical sociologist has characterized the "clinical mentality" as follows: (1) Action-oriented—the physician believes that he has to solve the problems that are brought to him and it is thus better to do something than to do nothing. (2) Self-reinforcing—the physician is biased toward believing that his or her intervention made the difference between success and failure, when in fact, that therapy might not have contributed to the outcome at all. This belief may have the desirable effect of influencing patients to respond favorably to a placebo, but it may also make the patient feel that his or her own body with its natural defenses against illness and injury was less important than it actually was in attaining a cure or improvement. This bias may also influence the physician to see improvement or cure where none has actually occurred—and as a result, to overestimate the value of his own decisions and intervention. (3) Emphasizing indeterminacy and uncertainty—since each individual's medical course may be different, medical outcomes can't be predicted and the physician assumes a certain responsibility for the outcome. If he or she alone assumes that responsibility, then he or she must also be entitled to assume responsibility for decision-making. Although Ed MacPhee was happy to leave all decision-making responsibility in his physician's hands, the inability of many patients to play a larger role in making decisions about their health and health care is a source of conflict between doctor and patient.

## Sources of Conflict in the Doctor-Patient Relationship

We are all aware of references to the "sacred doctor-patient relationship." But it is important to distinguish that almost mythical relationship from what one can expect realistically. The mythical doctor-patient relationship is free of conflict; the real one, potentially full of conflict. The mythical doctor-patient relationship is supposed to be perfect: the doctor understands all the patient's concerns, needs, and fears, and responds in such a way that the patient is not only cured, but is enriched by the totally satisfying contact he has had with the physician. The cost of maintaining this myth can be substantial when either patient or physician fails to foresee potential conflicts and neither person works to overcome the potential problems.

Even before his first contact with the health care system, the patient faces a double bind: he is expected to assess his own condition (and not bring trivial complaints to the physician's attention), but at the same time he is expected to leave diagnosis and prognosis in the hands of the physician. Better-informed patients, like Jeanne McLaughlin, might generate even more conflict. Another source of conflict lies in the fundamental assymetry in the patient's and physician's views of a particular illness: the patient may see a threat to his or her health as the most important thing in the world. But the physician—forced to allocate time among many patients competing for attention—may see that same threat as "just another case of disease 64." The patient may also view his problem as unique and be offended by the physician who offers an explanation based on a statistical probability. Treatment based on statistical likelihoods may be even more difficult to accept when the patient realizes that medical knowledge is incomplete and that physicians are sometimes wrong.

The natural anxiety surrounding threats to one's health or life may also lead a patient to want a physician to be totally selfless, totally dedicated, and extremely incapable of error. But these expectations are not likely to be fulfilled. Jenny Monroe came right out and said what was on her mind when she asked her physician if he ever made mistakes. Jenny's mother, on the other hand, was reluctant to question the physician, afraid that he might find the questions of an ordinary mother ridiculous. In her mind, at least, the physician was not human enough to question. It is hard to know whether Mrs. Monroe was intimidated by the image of the doctor she wished for, or whether that physician had actually acted in ways to suggest that her questions were ridiculous.

In some instances, the distance between physician and patient may reflect a cultural distance created by the elevated socioeconomic status of physicians in our culture. This difference in physicians' incomes, status, and educational level may engender resentment, as well as intimidation or fear. Finally, conflict very commonly arises when the patient's desire for certainty runs up against the physician's view that the course of a disease is inherently uncertain, the future unpredictable.

### Tools of Control in the Doctor-Patient Relationship

Doctor and patient both have means of asserting control in their encounters. Physicians can use their social status, training, or education to intimidate patients. They have an advantage in possessing greater knowledge about the body and health care, while most individuals are consumers of health care only rarely and know very little about it. Patients also lack information with which they might judge a physician's competence. Physicians can further intimidate patients and obscure specific issues by resorting to the use of jargon, or using Greek or Latin instead of English. Physicians can label something an "emergency," thereby unilaterally assigning priority to a problem that may be urgent but relatively unimportant. Physicians keep their clothes on, while patients take theirs off. Physicians stand up, while patients lie down. Physicians control the appointment schedule and have the power to keep patients waiting. Physicians also control referrals to specialists and access to medical resources. Finally, the physician has the power to certify who is ill and who a malingerer; who is temporarily insane and who the coldly calculating criminal.

Patients have their own means of asserting control. To begin with, they need not seek medical care. They can refuse to pay, seek second opinions, or shop for a doctor they do like. They can minimize or exaggerate symptoms or give misinformation. They can refuse to comply with the doctor's orders. And they can intimidate through threats of malpractice litigation.

With so many tools of control available to both parties in the encounter, there are many potential obstacles to a desired outcome. On the other hand, when each party recognizes the importance and power of the other, both may work together to facilitate the desired outcome. Some observers have described the optimal process as one of "negotiation." The key to the success of this negotiation lies in effective communication between doctor and patient.

### Communication in the Doctor-Patient Relationship

Communication in the doctor-patient encounter is not always direct, explicit, or acknowledged. Nor is it limited to spoken words: people communicate through body language, dress, props, and silence. Even the arrangement of furniture within an office may communicate a clear notion of how the patient is expected to relate to the physician. Many modes may be employed, but to be effective, communication must satisfy three requirements. First, the communicator must *desire* to transmit information accurately. This desire can be obstructed by other needs and wishes, some conscious, others not. For example, a patient's desire to transmit information may be clouded by fears, by a desire to avoid certain stigmata, or by an eagerness to please the physician. Ed MacPhee deliberately chose not to communicate to his surgeon any information about his previous experience with alcohol or psychiatric illness. The physician must also want to communicate, but he, too, may experience conflicting feelings or needs. He may feel, for example, that he does not have time to communicate, or he may mistakenly believe that the patient is either unable to comprehend or that the patient understands more than he actually does. At times, his desire to communicate may conflict with his wish to keep the patient ignorant as a way of maintaining professional dominance.

The second element of effective communication is the *ability* to transmit information. This ability requires that the sender and recipient of the information share a common language and a common culture. Sandy Heywood, for example, felt that she understood almost nothing that her doctors said to her during the first few months of her hospitalization; her doctors, in turn, found it hard to understand what they termed her "street lingo." When Meg Crissara was told that her husband had had a vascular occlusion, she barely reacted: she did not know what it meant. The ability of doctors and patients to communicate effectively may be further limited when they do not share a common experience. How does a physician convey to a patient what it means for a given operation to have, say, a 5 percent risk of death? How might Meg Crissara have understood what Joel's physicians meant when they said he would have an 80 percent recovery? Jenny Monroe's mother was told that the risk of Jenny's dying from general anesthesia was 1 in 10,000, but there was little in her prior experience to help her deal with such numbers. On the other hand, does the physician understand what it's like to be told that one's spouse has just had a stroke? Dr. Caplan's willingness to stay with Meg after he told her that her husband had just had a stroke indicates that Dr. Caplan did appreciate what it might mean to Meg, even though his experience as a physician taking care of stroke patients was quite different from the experience Meg was to have. A difference in experience need not pose an insurmountable barrier to effective communication.

The third requirement for effective communication is that the listener be *receptive.* Physicians may be less than totally receptive when they exercise selective attention, listening only to what they consider important to making a diagnosis or listening only to what they have time to hear. Patients, on the other hand, may not hear what is said because of their anxiety or their desire to deny what is said while waiting for the answer they want to hear.

Failure to satisfy any of these requirements for effective communication—desire and ability to transmit information on the part of the speaker and receptivity on the part of the listener—will limit the value of any doctor-patient interaction and may result in persistent misunderstanding. Why, for example, didn't Sandy Heywood know that she would no longer urinate after her kidneys were removed? Was it that her physician never mentioned it? Was it mentioned in language she did not understand? Or was she just not ready to hear it when she was told?

There are no easy answers to these problems that illness presents to patients, families, and health care workers. I have tried to present some of these issues in a way that may make them easier to discuss, believing that recognizing and discussing them is the necessary beginning for their solution.